D1418930

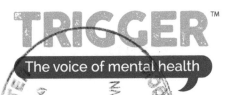

The voice of mental health

www.triggerpublishing.com

Thank you for purchasing this book.
You are making an incredible difference.

Proceeds from all Trigger books go directly to
The Shaw Mind Foundation, a global charity that focuses
entirely on mental health. To find out more about
The Shaw Mind Foundation visit,
www.shawmindfoundation.org

MISSION STATEMENT

Our goal is to make help and support available for every
single person in society, from all walks of life.
We will never stop offering hope. These are our promises.

Trigger and The Shaw Mind Foundation

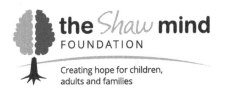

the *Shaw* mind
FOUNDATION

Creating hope for children,
adults and families

CONTENTS

INTRODUCTION

'Men don't get depressed.' Or at least that's what people had always told me. 'Boys don't cry,' the teachers said. 'Pull yourself together,' the blokes in the pub would say. 'Count your blessings and get on with your life.'

Well, I counted my blessings. And I didn't have anything to worry about. A good income, a wonderfully supportive wife, and a beautiful baby boy. We had a nice house, we took some wonderful holidays ... so why did I feel like my life was falling apart?

I'd been taught to take on life like a man, so when our son was born by emergency caesarean, I tried to tough it out. When my wife got depressed after the birth, I tried to hide my feelings and carry on. And then, when I started to experience symptoms of postnatal depression, I tried to ignore it. I tried to drink my PND under the table. Because I was a man.

I always thought my strength would protect me, but in the end, my depression was so much stronger.

I didn't know where my depression came from. I was just a normal working bloke. I was just like everyone else. And that's the point. Depression isn't selective. It doesn't pick and choose who it wants. It can hit any of us, at any time of our lives. And it hit me, hard.

This isn't just my story. It's the story of a movement for greater understanding of men's mental health issues – and men's experience of postnatal depression that has grown and grown. Above all, it is the story of how one little family came through depression, and, against all the odds, survived. This is a story made possible by, and dedicated to, my family – to Michelle and Ethan.

CHAPTER 1

I was born in August 1974, and raised in a beautiful village in the South Wales Valleys called Ogmore Vale (Cwm Ogwr in Welsh), about nine miles from the town of Bridgend.

It was a time of social unrest in the UK: inflation was rising, the miners' strike was dragging on, and the government was in a mess. The world my parents had known – with all its old certainties – was changing fast.

The coal mines in South Wales were beginning to close. By the eighties, they'd all be gone. That had (and still has) a huge impact on our community. Families started moving away from the valley to work. My generation became the first generation that didn't have to work underground for a living.

My dad was one of the last miners in South Wales. He left school at 15, and went straight down the mines, where he worked as a fitter and kept the machinery running, right down there at the pit bottom. He toiled away in that hidden world for the next 29 years, until he finished at the Nantgarw pit in 1987, one of the last mines in Wales to be closed. Dad couldn't afford to just idle the rest of his days away, and his pride wouldn't have let him, so he carried on working as a postman until he retired at 65. Before I was born, my mam worked as a mental health nurse, and later got a job working in a local garage.

Both of my parents were very hard-working and between them hardly ever had any time off. I can't remember them ever moaning about their jobs, but I always felt like neither of them were appreciated for their hard work, especially Mam during her 25 years at the garage.

I was an only child, but I don't ever remember being lonely. I was never inside long enough to watch television or mope around being bored like some children did. I played with my grandparents, who I loved very much, and they loved me right back. In a time where there was very little money, they provided me with enough so that I was never bored.

It may not sound like the best place to grow up, and times were hard for the whole community, but I'm proud of my heritage. I am a Valley boy born and bred. In fine weather, which I admit can be a rarity down here, I often sit and relax on the Bwlch Mountain. You can see for miles along the stunning South Wales coastline and across the Bristol Channel. Sometimes, when I'm feeling down, I go there, to drink in all that natural beauty, and remind myself of the life that I am so grateful for.

I was loved by my family, and I made friends at school, but life wasn't always easy. Whenever I spoke, I would mumble. Or the words would come out too fast, and I'd trip over my tongue. People could barely understand me. And it would just get worse if they asked me to repeat myself. Even to this day, when I get excited, I have a tendency to run through my words, sentences crashing into one another inside my mouth. I can see the looks of confusion in people's faces when they try to understand what I'm saying, and it takes me right back to my childhood, right back to when it was really bad.

By age eight, I was going to a private clinic each week, and it was all paid for by the school. If it hadn't been for them, I doubt I would have ever had the help I needed. I had to learn how to get past it. I wanted to be able to speak so that people could understand what I was saying. The speech and language therapists encouraged me to sit still, slow down and really think about what I was saying. But it didn't come easily to me. I was young and full of restless energy, and sometimes, I'd get fed up with it all. It wasn't enough for me to just sit down and think about what I was saying; I wanted something to *do.* But they just carried on telling me to try to slow down.

I can't remember how many lessons I ended up having, but I do remember it wasn't a quick fix. It felt like I carried on suffering with it for a long time. So, in the end, I found my own ways of dealing with it by treating it like it was all a bit of a joke. That Valleys boy who tried to make people laugh as a way of hiding from his fears is still a big part of me.

So I smiled and I laughed and "kept on carrying on". But inside, I knew there was something deeply wrong with me. I often felt upset. It felt like there was nothing I could do to change who I was or what I was. There was no hiding from it in class and I started avoiding certain words because I didn't want people to laugh at me. When the jokes dried up, I started to get quieter.

The other kids at school all seemed so happy, so carefree, so *normal*, but I couldn't get past my worries. As my anxiety about school grew, I started to wet the bed. Or I would lie there, unable to sleep, thinking about how much I didn't want to go to school the next day. I hated the smell of the classroom, the feel of the wooden desk with the ink pot, the way the teachers treated us. I remember them shouting at us, their faces screwed up in anger. Sometimes they'd throw blackboard dusters; sometimes they'd actually slap us. To be hit, and shouted at, and told to keep still by people that were so scary, that were so mean, that were so callous ... I thought it was normal. I suppose, back then, it was normal. But looking back, it was terrifying that things like that were allowed to happen.

It wasn't the entire school that I hated; I had some great friends in primary school, and I was never bullied in the playground. But as soon as I was in class, I wanted to escape. I was so terrified of being shouted at that I just couldn't take anything in. So, if the teachers asked me anything, I would freeze, and then they would shout at me again. It was like being trapped in a vicious cycle with no way out.

Whenever I got bored in class, which was a lot of the time, I couldn't stop my mind from wandering, especially when I was doing something hard, like writing. I used to drift off and end up doing a really rushed job so that I could do something else that made me feel better. To this day, I still do that. I run away from my difficulties. People call it procrastination, but I just call it coping.

I guess it was because of these school anxieties that I was described as a 'slow learner' on all of my reports. Then I had to go and have "special lessons" for reading with a teacher called Mrs Goode. I hated being placed in that class. It was for stupid people, and I wasn't one of them. I resisted Mrs Goode at first, but slowly, she turned me around. Hearing her slow and melodic voice would calm me, and as I sat with her, my reading began to progress so much faster than it had before.

There are some teachers who we will remember from school for all the hatred they threw our way, and there are some teachers who we remember because they helped us more than they will ever know … teachers like Mrs Goode. I'll never forget her for as long as I live.

Now, because I lived in Wales, it rained. It rained a lot. When I think back to primary school, it seemed like the rain came lashing down at us every day. Maybe once I would have thought that God was punishing us again for the sins we had committed.

I hated the rain so much, because when it rained it meant we had to stay in the classroom, and I would get more and more fidgety and anxious. Like a wound-up toy, I needed to be let loose. I felt like I had to escape the classroom I was stuck in. But the teachers never let us out, not even for a second. And that's when things started to change … I started playing games with the other kids, and quite soon they were looking to me for ideas for more games. It turns out I was the one who had the best ideas. Maybe all of that time feeling trapped in class had made my imagination soar.

I was proud of my creativity. As well as the games that I would think up whenever me and my friends were in need of fun, I started to use my creativity in class. Any time the teacher gave us a problem, I would begin to look at it in a different way from other people. Instead of hitting it head on, I would try to see it from different angles, to try to understand the problem from every single perspective possible. I never wanted to do things the way the teacher wanted; I needed to do things my own way. But the problem was that I got so wrapped up in thinking about the problem that if a teacher asked me another question, I couldn't say anything. And then I would get in trouble all over again, for not listening.

But despite all the trouble I was in, I was never particularly naughty in class. A bit of a daydreamer yes, but never cheeky. I was raised to treat my elders with respect. I can't ever imagine saying something bad to my parents or my grandparents! I was raised to be a good boy, and that's what I was in school ... well, a good boy with a tendency not to pay attention ...

But it's only now, all these years later, that I understand where all my behaviours came from. The way I was easily distracted, the lack of attention and focus, the daydreaming. It all made so much sense to me once I began to learn more about what I had. I didn't know it then, but I had Attention deficit hyperactivity disorder (ADHD).

Looking back, I wish that there had been more education for my teachers regarding mental health, especially ADHD. I don't feel any anger, or hatred, or bitterness towards my teachers; I know it wasn't their fault – they were simply brought up in a different world. I can't expect them to know that which was not taught to them. But even now, things aren't as good as they should be, and that is something that makes me really angry.

Outside of school, there was one thing that really helped me: The Wyndham Boys and Girls Club. It was only open for boys back in the eighties, but I'm glad it's open for everyone now. Back then, Stan 'The Man' Norris volunteered for children in the valley – a complete and utter valley legend!

It was Stan who gave me the push to better myself. He often pushed me to go to tournaments and inspired me in ways my teachers never did. Thanks to his encouragement, I entered an under-sixteens' pool tournament and won. I was the British Champion, and my photograph was put on display at the club and in the school.

I hadn't ever imagined that I'd have won anything, or excelled at anything. The anxious boy was still there, but was slowly getting more confident. I was so proud when we collected our awards in a full house at the local club. And it gave me the confidence to think that I could do more things with my life, if I tried hard enough.

Looking back now, it was the Boys Club that gave me the confidence I needed, the confidence that I had lost with my mumbling, and my terror of the teachers. Without being too arrogant, I was pretty good at most sports, and so it was nice to have someone see that in me and tell me I was doing well. It sounds like such a small thing, but as a child, it was everything that I needed.

Time passed quickly for me after primary school. I made new friends at secondary school. I wasn't mumbling any more, but I was still going through the motions in class, and I never really thought about pursuing an education beyond that. I never felt I was good enough in school. No one ever made me feel like I could amount to anything.

The only thing I wanted to do when I left school was to get a job and earn my own money so that I could do all the things I wanted. I had seen my parents work hard, and I wanted to follow in their footsteps.

I was already looking far ahead, counting the days until I could leave.

CHAPTER 2

Our memories make us, don't they? There will always be things that we look back on with joy and happiness, but for me, it's the things I remember with a sense of shame or embarrassment that have left the deepest impression. My childhood is filled with these moments, from the embarrassment of being caught in a lie, to being in trouble with my teachers ... but there is one thing that I will never forget, and always regret.

When I was ten, I had my first experience of alcohol. Stupidly young, I know, but it was just the way of the world back then. It was New Year's Eve and it seemed like *everyone* was drinking. I was allowed to go out with my older friends, and then we ended up walking the streets. And someone passed me a bottle – I had no idea what was in it, but that didn't even matter. I just knew I had to drink it because if I didn't, everyone would think I was a wimp. Even at age ten, I knew I couldn't lose face like that. In a world where men were men, I had a reputation to build. So I put it to my lips and took a gulp, and then another, and another ...

... And then all I remember after that is lying on the sofa at home, feeling a whole new kind of sick. It was like my body was punishing me for drinking. I felt like death. For days after that, I thought I'd never, ever drink again.

And I didn't. Well, not for a few years anyway. I waited until I was 13 years old before I really started drinking regularly. My drinking buddies were all older than me, so there was no way they were going to allow me to drink a few cokes. It was pints all the way. But the more I drank, the calmer I felt. It was as if all that tension I'd had at school just drained away.

At weekends, big groups of us would head out to parties, or, in desperation, hang around bus stops. I quickly became the person known in the group for taking things too far and getting totally off my head. I was the one people talked about: 'Oh did you hear what Mark did last night?' And I liked that. So I'd go even further the next time. I wanted people to go on talking about me.

I left school at 15 without a single qualification to my name. But they couldn't have made me stay a day longer than I had to. By now, I was drinking to professional standards! I was hiding away from responsibilities; relying on the drink. I didn't want to let go of it. And it didn't want to let go of me.

I did a few jobs here and there, small things that didn't pay very much, until I started to work on a government youth training scheme as a bricklayer.

The local kids didn't have the same job security generations of young men had had in the Valleys. We didn't have a working identity. The mines were closed. We had to find something else. I thought being a bricklayer would give me a tribe – a gang of mates who would be there for each other, through thick and thin. I even thought that could be my entire working life all mapped out. But all we ever seemed to do was talk about laying bricks, and never seemed to actually do any bricklaying, so I began to look for other work. There were still jobs out there then, despite the closure of the mines, and I soon found a job working at a local factory.

It wasn't perfect. I didn't expect perfect, but I did expect to get some respect. My manager seemed to have a problem with everyone who worked there, including me. He would ask me to do overtime, but only on his terms. He'd call me into his office, just so he could order me around. I never understood why he did this. We already knew that he had the power over us – he was our manager – but he clearly never wanted to let us forget it.

Life was starting to move in a different direction. For the first time in my life, I had money – and I wasn't afraid to spend it! I was 16 years old, and life outside of work was easy. I stopped going to the Boys Club, stopped playing football, and started partying. Monday to Thursday at the factory was followed by a long weekend of drinking to excess. I sobered up for Monday morning, and then did it all over again.

The rave scene was really taking off and I jumped in, feet first. It was all about the music, the parties and the excess. I had a completely different set of friends, and they were all into it. They'd invite me out to parties and nightclubs, and I never said no. It was through them that I enjoyed so much new music, and so many new experiences. I felt so alive whenever I was with them.

I started smoking too. I'd always hated being around smokers as a kid, and I never, ever thought I'd be a smoker, but it was getting harder to say no to all those new experiences. So there I was, buying packet after packet of cigarettes, along with everyone else. I even moved on to smoking pot; what would my 10-year-old self have thought of older Mark? Would he even have recognised the man I was turning into?

I carried on working in the factory, and I carried on drinking. I was earning more money than I ever had, and I loved going clubbing and getting completely wasted. I was having the time of my life. Or at least, I thought I was. As the drinking got worse, I started having blackouts. I'd wake up after another skin-full, not remembering a single thing I'd done the night before. I used to tell myself it was fine: after all, if I didn't remember, then I couldn't regret whatever I'd done. I would sometimes wake up in gutters, or just lying in the street, without any knowledge of how I had gotten there in the first place.

Sometimes I'd wake up in a police cell. I never knew how I'd got there. At least once, I nearly died after choking on my own vomit.

The memories were hazy then; they're even more blurred with time now, but there are little flashes of the things that I did, still there, in the back of my mind. So why did I do it? Why did I carry on drinking?

I liked being around my friends. I still liked impressing them. But more than anything, I needed the confidence I only got from drinking.

When I wasn't with my friends, I often felt low. I hated that. I hated feeling so down. Whenever I was by myself, I'd suddenly start feeling anxious about my life, about the shape it had become. I didn't know where I was going, or what I was supposed to do with my life. And in between the drinking, those questions really started to bother me.

As I approached the end of my teenage years, these questions came up more and more. I was completely lost inside. I didn't have a single idea about what I wanted to do with my life. All I did during the working week was look forward to the end of it. And then at the weekend, I'd get completely wrecked all over again. And on and on it went.

I wanted to find out who I really was, underneath it all. But I couldn't face up to those thoughts alone. When I came back from work, I struggled because then I really was on my own. There was no one around me, and I needed people to talk to. So I started to buy notepads to write down ideas of what I could do with my time. I thought that I could go and see live bands, or try activities I had never done before. I dreamt of travelling ... maybe one day I could see the world. I bought countless notepads, scribbling down ideas onto the pages, ticking them off whenever I could. It filled the time when I was left alone with my thoughts.

I had done such a good job of fitting in that it took me a while to realise there were aspects of me that were different to other people. I found it hard to concentrate on just one thing, and I was always distracted. My mind was always all over the place, which meant it could take ages to find my keys or my wallet. It was like I wasn't always in control of my mind. It was starting to feel a lot like school all over again.

At first, I had enjoyed getting my own money and being able to spend it on things that I wanted. But as time passed and as I spent more and more weeks, and months, and years there, I began to hate Monday mornings. On Sunday nights, I'd lie awake, staring up at the ceiling, dreading waking up in the morning and having to go to work. It was just like all those years at school, all over again.

The turning point came when my grandfather was taken into hospital. The doctors told us that it was only a matter of time. The man who had done so much for me growing up was dying. We all stayed with him until the end. With his family all around him, he took his final breath, and then his heart stopped beating.

Nights like this, they can teach a person a lot. I felt so connected to my own dad that night. I learnt a lot about what it means to be a father, about what it means to be a son, and about the special relationship that only a father and son can have. I look back on that night from time to time, especially now that I have my own son. I can only hope that one day he will feel that same bond with me too.

I saw my father cry when my grandfather died. It was the first and only time I had ever seen him cry. And I cried alongside him. I couldn't stop thinking of all the time my grandfather and I had spent together when I was younger, when he would play with me. I think I spent more time with him than I did my own parents, and I loved him so much.

I can still feel the pain of losing him, even now. And that fear of losing someone close to me never quite went away.

They say life goes on. So, next morning, I was still expected to go into work. But the very thought of it, after everything that had happened, just made me want to cry even more. And after staying up all night, I knew that it would be dangerous for me to work with machinery.

So I walked into the office and explained the situation to my boss, thinking he'd understand. To my complete and utter disbelief, he just told me to get to work. I was shocked. I just stared at him, and I knew then that he didn't care about me at all. None of them did. I couldn't believe his callousness; it was like a scene from a film. I knew then that I was easily replaceable. I was just a number to him, nothing more. So, cut to the end scene: I walked away from them and never looked back.

After nearly six years working there, it all came down to this single moment. I felt as if my eyes had finally been opened to what a soul-sucking place it was. Thank God it didn't take me another 10, 20, 30 years to walk away.

I still knew that I wanted my life to have a purpose. I wanted more than just sitting on a factory production line. I wanted something to give my life some meaning. I loved working with the people there, and still have some incredible friends from those days, but I hated the place and the rules.

I was young, and I had a good long stretch of work on my CV, so getting another job was pretty easy. I hadn't given up on my dreams just yet. Every time I opened my notebook I'd remind myself of my biggest ambition: to travel the world. So I started saving up straightaway.

Other people weren't keen on the idea. My mother was worried about me. But I knew it was something that I needed to do for myself. I told her it was the right time. I didn't want to just stay in this small part of the world, I wanted to see as much of it as possible. I understood why my mother was scared: I was doing things that no one in my family had ever done before. But I knew I couldn't tie myself down to a dead-end job and waste my life away, like so many people did where I lived.

I'd been lucky enough to go abroad on holidays, and it had given me an itch for travel that I had to scratch. I was young, with no responsibilities, and I knew that if I didn't grab that opportunity there and then, I never would.

I decided then that I wasn't going to hang around. I wasn't going to waste any opportunity to live my life the way I wanted. So I bought my ticket and went by train around Europe. I started in Holland, travelled to Germany and Switzerland, and then onto Spain, Monaco and Greece. I walked around these countries and cities and places, all of them so different from my home in the Valleys. I drank it all in; the lights and the colours, the people and the accents, the food and the sights. I loved it all so much, and every time I moved on from one place to another I felt the pain of leaving those new experiences behind me. I loved everything about it. Not just the thrill of the adventure, but the way it opened my eyes to a wider world.

My friends back home thought that I was completely crazy to give up my job, just to go travelling. They were convinced that I would never get a job again. But within a couple of weeks of returning, I had another full-time job. I had a good attitude, and jobs were easy enough to find – if you didn't think too hard about what you were doing. I just needed to work and get money so that I could do all the things I wanted to do.

But coming home was tough. I'd quit the job I hated, and had an amazing experience, but life was just the same when I got back. All the same frustrations crept back. All the same worries. All the drinking ...

Drinking became an essential part of me, and I didn't know anything else. I would feel part of something whenever I drank. Like I belonged. But I only liked to drink with people who would get as drunk as me, or even worse. I saw people losing their lives to alcohol, and I could have gone the same way; I just wasn't ready to face the truth back then. So I surrounded myself with people who had it just as bad as I did.

The booze was fun. But I knew I was hiding from myself. Drinking helped me keep everything locked up deep inside. But it was getting worse. Sometimes when I was drinking and I blacked out, I would wake up with a woman I couldn't remember from the night before. And I wouldn't always know if I had worn a condom. It would make me feel sick with worry the next day. I would always phone my friends to see how much I'd embarrassed myself. And then I would hate myself for it, and give in to the depression, until the weekend came around again.

In 1995, at the age of 22, having been living this life for seven years, I entered a relationship with a girl the same age as me. I wondered if being responsible for someone else would change how I lived my life. But looking back now, I know that I wasn't ready to settle down. I wanted fun. And more fun. With a little bit of extra fun on the side. It didn't matter how I was going to find it, or who I had to push aside to get it.

But a lifestyle like that takes its toll. By the time 1996 rolled around, I was severely underweight and depressed. I remember my close friends telling me over and over again about how bad I looked. They said that it was because of my girlfriend. It's true the relationship wasn't working, but it was the partying that was doing the damage. It felt like we were holding each other back, and, as usual, the drinking was my way of coping with that. I ended it with her soon afterwards.

I was starting to feel as if the people around me were saying bad things about me. I didn't know if it was the truth or just paranoia. But I knew I was doing some serious damage to my body, and I started to feel bad about the way I was living my life. I was hardly eating anything, and my partying lifestyle was getting out of control. I had gained a police record for being drunk and disorderly and causing an affray. If I wanted to destroy my future job prospects, I was doing a pretty good job of it. Something had to change.

As luck would have it, an advert came up in a national newspaper for jobs in Spain, and the interviews were being held in London. I took my father with me to make sure that I didn't do anything stupid, but it's clear as day to me now that I could have turned up dressed in anything I wanted; I still would have got the job. And that job was selling timeshares in Spain with an organisation that, I was soon to find out, was run by gangsters.

That word might conjure up an image of men dressed in black suits with hats and guns, but that wasn't the type of gangster that ran this company. No, these were what I like to call "mainstream gangsters", an entirely different breed of men. They were the type of people who would sell an Icelandic timeshare to an Eskimo. I did my time out there, tried to be as ethical as I could and then hightailed it out of there.

It wasn't all bad. That job gave me the confidence to sell. And it turned out that I was good at it. Unsurprisingly, for someone who likes to talk so much and is as friendly as I am, the job came very naturally to me. So I went back home, armed with the skills and the savvy to land myself a job in sales. As a sales rep, I had to wear some sharp suits, which I loved. And then there was the money. If you were good at your job, there was a whole lot of money. And I was very good at my job.

I couldn't believe that only a few years earlier, I'd been working in that awful factory and dreaming of driving the manager's cars. But now, I had a company car, and was earning three to four times my old weekly wage. The hours were better, and I was free from the daily grind of clocking on. It seemed like a dream come true.

My confidence was growing, and for the first time in my life I learnt how to listen to people more effectively. I learnt that I could be anything that I wanted to be in that job. I loved being around people from different walks of life, who all helped me see the world in so many different ways. I was in a different circle now. At times, my old life and my old friends seemed a very long way away.

But though I loved my job, there was still something missing, and after months of being single, I started to wonder about the possibility of seeing someone else. I might have been enjoying myself, but I wanted someone to enjoy things with.

And, as life would have it, I was about to find the woman who was going to become my rock.

CHAPTER 3

It was the weekend. I was back in Bridgend. Back with my old friends, back in all the old places. The same old pubs and clubs ...

I saw her as soon as we got inside. I was completely side-tracked by her big, blue eyes. She was so strikingly beautiful that I just couldn't stop staring at her from across the floor, trying to gather the nerves to speak to her. Somehow, I managed to walk over, say all the right words in all the right places, and ask her to dance.

This was one of those rare moments where the world seemed to just work for me. I hadn't gone in planning to meet anyone; it was just another day of going out and getting drunk. But there she was, and the world was pushing us together.

And after we danced, we went our separate ways. I remember thinking that there was no way I would ever see her again. Over the following ten months, I just filled my life with things so that I didn't stop to think about anything else.

It was after a holiday in Turkey with the boys that I felt the world working for me again. They all wanted to head straight out to a club in the Rhondda Valleys, a stone's throw away from where I lived. I was jet-lagged and all I wanted to do was sleep, but I didn't take much convincing; I never did. And within the hour, I was back at the bar. And it wasn't long before I noticed someone in the corner of the club sitting with her friends. I recognised her straightaway, though I couldn't remember where from. I had to go over and talk to her ...

She told me that her name was Michelle, and, suddenly, I had my lightbulb moment. This was the same girl I had met ten months ago in that nightclub in Bridgend! Sadly, Michelle didn't recognise me – maybe I hadn't made as big an impression on her as she obviously had on me! But I soon got over that, and asked her to dance with me. This time, I wasn't going to let her get away quite so easily. So, before I left, I made sure she had my address and phone number. She was just about to head off on holiday with the girls, but she promised she'd send me a postcard and ask me to meet up again.

After that night with Michelle, I was looking for a postcard every single day. But it wasn't until Michelle was nearly home that it finally arrived.

Within a few days of that postcard, we started seeing each other every week. Michelle was busy taking a business studies course at university, but we always made time to see one another, even if it was just one day a week.

I realised that I started to feel a closer connection to Michelle than I'd ever felt with anyone else. I found that I wanted to see her more and more, that every few days wasn't enough. I wanted to be with her as much as possible. I stopped hanging out with my friends as much, stopped drinking so much during the nights and the weekends, and found that I was happier for it. I know it made Michelle happier too.

Pretty soon, the relationship started moving fast. I met her family, and soon after that we went on our first holiday to Jamaica with friends. I remember we had a lot of good times there, with my best mate, Elwood. I was falling fast and I was falling deep. Pretty soon, I knew that I wanted nothing more than to spend the rest of my life with her.

After we came back from the holiday, Michelle went straight back to university and passed her degree. She was holding down three jobs as well as studying, and still managed to get a 2.2, which was incredible. I had never felt so proud of another person's achievements, and I was so happy for her.

When I saw Michelle in her cap and gown getting her degree, I was just in awe of what was happening. I was so glad to have been invited along with her parents. And I just knew, looking at her up there along with all the rest of her class, that this was the woman I was going to spend the rest of my life with.

One of the reasons why I found myself so taken with Michelle was her independence. She loved going out with her friends, just as much as I enjoyed going out with mine. I wanted to spend every second of my time with her, and although we'd moved in with my parents, I knew that it was important for each of us to have our own space. I never wanted Michelle to feel like I was trying to control her in any way. But there was one thing of mine that Michelle wanted to control: my drinking.

Michelle hated my drinking. And she hated it when I tried to get her to go drinking with me. I would try to keep her out with me as long as possible, and I never wanted to go home when she said she'd had enough. She told me I became a different person when I drank. That it was like the drink taking me over. I would always come up with excuses to have more and more, and then that would cause arguments.

Going out without her was worse. I'd leave the house, saying I'd be back in an hour, but as soon as the alcohol touched my lips, it was as though Michelle didn't exist. I'd forget that she was in the house waiting for me, and because there were no mobile phones around, she had no way of knowing where I was, how late I would be, or if I was even on my way back.

Even though she didn't like my drinking, we continued to grow stronger and stronger as a couple. Soon, Michelle moved in with me, and she began to see my drinking in the house for the first time. She would drink when she was out with her friends. She wouldn't have drunk at home, alone. But I didn't care if I was in company, or on my own; I would get pissed and then fall asleep in the sofa, or try to make it up to bed and fall asleep in the bath.

Michelle worried that in my drunkenness I would leave the cooker on and burn the entire house down, or that I'd cut myself trying to make food, or leave the front door open. I never did, but I carried on giving her cause to worry.

Somehow, I was still holding my adult life together and functioning in my job. I was still able to get up on time and go to work. I wasn't living the full partying lifestyle any more, but I was still on the cigarettes and the booze. Perhaps I didn't know it then, but I needed them to help me get by in my job. Working for sales commissions was tough, and sometimes my mind would just get too loud. It was easier if I didn't let myself think too hard about anything – and the drinking let me do that. It helped the negative thoughts and voices disappear.

We still argued about it. I didn't think my drinking was that bad. I just thought it was something everyone did, and that I was just fitting in. But Michelle knew I was drinking far more than other people. The blackouts were getting more regular and lasting far longer. Some days after a heavy weekend, I could hardly remember anything. Even if I didn't see my friends, I'd just get smashed on the weekends by myself.

I don't think that I was a horrible drunk. I never got angry at her, or threatened to hit her. But I would call her boring if she wanted to go home early, or if she tried to tell me I was drinking too much. She was right. The drink did take me over. It did change me. And I hated waking up the next morning, not knowing what I'd said to her the night before.

Drunk or sober, I adored Michelle's company. She was filled with warmth and love, and I just wanted to be with her. It was easy to imagine building our future together, with our own home and our own little family. And the more I thought about it, the more I wanted it.

After finishing university, Michelle started a new role in one of the big utilities companies, where she went on to coach new staff and run a target-driven team. It was pressurised work, and she had to deal with daily grievances, but Michelle never, ever complained about her workload. It meant we were bringing in a very good amount of money together. On the weekends, at Michelle's request, we started to go to restaurants and the theatre. Thanks to Michelle, I started to do things I had never done before, and I loved it. I started to look at things a little differently, even started to enjoy my work a bit more. I rose higher and higher in the company, and I worked hard to make it happen because it meant that I had more money to save for us, for our future.

We loved living with my parents, and my parents began to see Michelle as their own daughter, but we knew it wasn't going to be forever. We were planning to find our own place, but there was something else I needed to do first ...

There are two things I remember about 31st December 1999. Talk of the "Y2K bug" was being whipped into a frenzy by the media. The computer systems were going to crash, they warned us, causing the world to grind to a halt! I imagined what the world might look like without all these systems in place, and how long it'd be before we all killed each other! But we slipped into a new millennium without a hitch. And that night, dressed as a pirate in front of hundreds of people, I knelt down on one knee and asked Michelle (in her Little Miss Muffet costume) to marry me.

Thankfully, Little Miss Muffet screamed, 'YES!'

It was the start of a good year. We both had great jobs, and very few outgoings while we were still at my parents. So we still managed to go on holiday, and we still managed to buy nice things for one another. It was all good, but I was still drinking, and Michelle still hated it. There were so many times when Michelle could have left me, but she didn't.

At its worst, I was drinking as much as three to four bottles of wine a night. Work was still tough, but there was more to it than that …

My nan died suddenly from a heart attack early that year, and it hit me hard. We had been incredibly close. Really, she was like a second mother to me. She had loved me so much, and I never thought I'd ever get that kind of love from anyone else in my life. I had struggled with losing my grandfather, and this reminded me of just how fragile life can be. How it can be snatched from you in a second.

To cope with the sorrow and the grief of her passing, I turned to drinking. Of course I did. I didn't want anyone to know how I was feeling, so I hid behind a bottle. I wanted to pretend like there was nothing wrong, but everywhere I looked I saw memories of her, I heard her voice in my head.

Michelle tried to help, but I just didn't know how to tell her what I was feeling. (It's been 20 years since my nan passed away and I still think of her nearly every day.)

Later that year, I was given the chance to move to the Midlands with my well-paid sales role. It was hard work, but my boss treated me well, and I felt comfortable working there. I felt like my opinion was important and that people cared about me. I had the time and the money to live my life the way that I wanted to.

But though I loved my job, the question remained: was I really going to leave my home for it? Was I going to take us away from everything we knew and start all over again?

It was around this time that Michelle wanted to fulfil her ambition of travelling around Australia. At first, I was completely against the idea. But then, I remembered the wanderlust I'd felt. I remembered what an amazing experience my trip to Europe had been, and I didn't want to stand in her way. She had been working hard and had earned a sabbatical. I knew my boss would give me the opportunity to take some time off too. And the more we thought about it, the more we thought we should do it as a couple, so we applied for a visa and by June, we were headed for Bali, Thailand, and then down under for a few months.

It was the best of times, and coming back didn't feel scary at all. It was time to start our new lives together in a place of our own. Time to get married.

CHAPTER 4

We'd saved and saved for a deposit for our house and finally, after what seemed like an eternity, we were ready to find a place of our own. The plan had been that Michelle was going to stay at my mum and dad's until her exams were over. Now, it was three years later!

We knew the house we wanted as soon as we saw it. It was close to my old school, and it just felt like the perfect place for us to start this next stage of our lives together. So we checked our budget, put in an offer, and moved in within weeks.

The neighbours were all friendly, and I already knew some of them from football or from work. I couldn't go anywhere without bumping into someone I knew – even in Australia, I bumped into a familiar face within days of getting off the plane.

Being together in our own home was amazing. There were times when we could have really used another bedroom, but we loved it there. We were finally living together and our wedding was coming up …

We got married in Cyprus on 26th May 2003 – the day my football team got promoted to the Premier League! A special day for two totally different reasons. (Funny how I remember things when football is involved.)

I'll never forget the sight of Michelle in her wedding dress. I was honestly smitten. She looked completely stunning. In that moment, I felt so lucky to be her husband.

We had a wonderful night. We drank and talked and totally ruled the karaoke machine, which cleared out most of the hotel. I felt so happy being surrounded by my friends and family, but I felt even better when Michelle and I left the throng to start our married life together. That day is ingrained on my mind. Truly, one of the best days of my life.

Being with Michelle that night, I knew I wanted a family. It was such a sudden realisation. I had never, ever thought about having children before. But I felt the rush of excitement of knowing that I really wanted kids. I wanted it more than anything. At the age of 28, I was ready to experience fatherhood. Some of my friends were already becoming fathers and they seemed so happy. There haven't been many times in my life that I have been 100% certain about something, but on this, I was completely committed.

We talked and talked about it, and we were both so excited at the thought of starting a family together. I hadn't expected it to happen quite so quickly, but within a few weeks, Michelle thought she might be pregnant.

We had already booked tickets for the cinema that night, and, in a bit of a daze, decided to go anyway. I don't think we remembered any of the film as we walked back to the car. I guess we were both so excited, so nervous, and so absolutely amazed that we were going to become parents. It felt real and unreal all at the same time.

It certainly took me a little while to process the information. But two positive pregnancy test results later, we were ready for our lives to change!

We told our parents as soon as we could. But we managed to wait just long enough to make sure the early stages of the pregnancy were going well. The news floored them at first. But I don't think I've ever seen them look happier.

Over the next few months, we just enjoyed the idea that the baby was coming. We didn't have any worries that we weren't ready for it. We were just high on the excitement of it all.

There are so many things that a new baby needs, and we wanted to make sure we were well prepared, so we were making changes, and saving money. I was making changes to myself too. After far too many years, I gave up smoking. Michelle had always been a fierce anti-smoker – but still managed to put up with me! But the arrival of a new baby changed things. Neither of us wanted the baby to be around someone who was smoking as much as I was. (Michelle had never let me smoke inside, so at least I didn't have to go outside in the cold to smoke any more!)

Some couples don't want to know whether they're going to have a boy or a girl until their baby is born, but we really wanted to know. Michelle had always told me that our first child was going to be a boy, and at the 20-week scan, we found out she was right. I couldn't believe it. I was so overjoyed. I'd always wanted a son, and I couldn't wait until I could start doing father–son things with him.

The excitement was so vivid. I could almost reach out and touch the future I could see in my mind. But after that huge high, I felt a little bit low. There was so much that could still go wrong, and I started to worry if the baby was going to be healthy. That was all that mattered to me.

We kept copies of the 20-week scan image, and I kept mine in my wallet throughout the time Michelle was pregnant. I must have showed that picture off so many times over the next few months, shoving it in the faces of everyone that I met. It was just amazing to me to be able to see a photo of the person that Michelle was growing inside her. A true miracle.

It seemed that things were going really well for Michelle and me. We had everything that we wanted: marriage, home, and a baby boy on the way.

As the weeks passed, nights out turned into nights in, watching DVDs and just curling up on the sofa together. Instead of going out drinking, we went to antenatal classes at the local hospital. But, if I'm honest, I learnt very little at those classes. Though we met a nice couple while we were there, I just wanted to get out of there as soon as possible. Maybe it was being back in a classroom environment that set me off. I found it hard to concentrate, and the more I worried about it, the worse it got. What if something went wrong at the birth and I didn't know what to do? What if I'd missed hearing some vital fact that could save my baby's life? What if I was a terrible father?

Later, I wished over and over again that I had listened more.

It wasn't because I wasn't interested; I just couldn't tell you anything the nurse had said to us. It was mostly about all the good things that would happen at the birth. She told us what the room would look like, and how to prepare ourselves for the day of the birth.

I do remember they showed us a birth on the television, which was incredible. I didn't know it at the time, but that would be the closest I would ever come to seeing a natural birth. If I'd known what a caesarean section (C-section) was, I would have wanted to see that being done too, as it would have been good preparation for what was about to come. But, of course, I didn't know that at the time.

At no point during the class was there any mention of birth trauma, emergency C-sections, or postnatal depression.

The last few weeks were such a drag: waiting, waiting, waiting, shopping for baby clothes, waiting, waiting, wallpapering, waiting ...

The waiting was really hard. And I was trying hard not to drink, but I could feel all the familiar cravings crawling in my head. Sometimes, I'd have a bottle of wine or two in the house, but never anything more than that. But I was good, and stayed home with Michelle the entire time. Well, almost ...

There was one time when I was the best man at my workmate's wedding. The usher and I went on a 24-hour bender, while Michelle sat at home, heavily pregnant, feeling on edge in case things started happening ahead of schedule – not exactly my best moment.

After that, I felt as if things changed. It wasn't just that I regretted it; I started to think that it was time to grow up. I knew I wanted to be the best father I could for our new family. I was already imagining it – picturing what it would be like to have a child, to hold him in my arms, to make him giggle and laugh at his silly old dad. One day soon I would be able to take *my son* to football. I started to plan it all out in my head, and I just wanted him to be born so we could start getting to know him.

But as I started planning, I started to worry more and more. I knew that we had to have enough money to raise him properly. I started thinking about my job. I was a good salesman, but the pressure never stopped, and I hated the days when I couldn't reach my targets. I felt trapped. I knew I couldn't leave: I had to keep on working hard, and keep on hitting those targets – the baby and Michelle would be depending on me.

I decided that we would need to make some more changes. We couldn't just jump on a plane and go travelling any more. We couldn't just buy things whenever we wanted, we couldn't just splash out on a night out at the theatre. We were going to have a baby to look after, and that was a big job.

Something else was worrying me too. Expectations for fatherhood had changed massively since it was my dad wondering how he was going to manage with a new baby in his life. These days, it's more involved, more inclusive, and there are far more things resting on the father's shoulders than ever before. When my father was younger, all that was expected was that the father went to work and provided for the family. But that didn't feel like it was going to be enough for me. I wanted to do all of that, of course, but I wanted to be around for my family and my child too.

I was going to be more involved in his care. I felt as if I had to do more, to *be* more than those who had come before me.

My father hadn't had the experience of watching my mother give birth to me. He had been told to stay at home and Mum had given birth alone in the hospital. Later, Dad phoned the ward to be told he had a son. It was how they did things back then. My grandparents were up in Liverpool, and they couldn't be there either. It sounded like such a lonely way to bring someone into the world, but Mum says it was a walk in the park! Back then, the community was like an extended family. Everyone rallied round and looked out for each other.

As I thought more about my child, I found myself thinking about my own father. How would I measure up to him? Had he been a good dad to me, or had he just done what was expected of him at the time? How do you measure that, anyway – what makes some people good dads?

I just knew that I wanted to be the best dad ever. I felt ready for fatherhood, for the challenge of it. I felt as if I had gone beyond living for the weekends and going out with my friends. I wanted something more now. I was ready to live for my family. And I was so sure we had done the right thing. I never for a second thought that we had made a mistake by choosing to have this baby.

We were lucky. Not long before our due date, some very good friends of ours lost their child around the 18-week mark. It was one of the hardest things we've done, watching our good friends go through something so traumatic, while we were so excited about Michelle's pregnancy. And inevitably, it made us worry about our own child, and about everything that could still go wrong. There were so many restless nights, so many moments of panic and stress, but as the weeks went by, the excitement started to build ...

Finally, November, and our due date, rolled around. We'd planned it all out in detail; Michelle's bags were all packed, and we were just waiting for her body to tell her it was ready. Because I was pretty much self-employed as a sales rep, I'd been able to plan a few weeks off, and we had set aside enough money to see us through the next few weeks.

When the time came, it felt special. If storming out of work had been one big movie scene, this was another. It's still so vivid in my mind: I was closing a sale in a supermarket, and was just saying goodbye to the customer when my phone started to ring ...

It was Michelle. She was completely calm, but asked me to come home. I think in my heart I knew that it was time. When I got there, she was having a cup of tea, just patiently waiting for me. We held back a little longer, just to make sure that it was really happening – and because Michelle didn't want to leave until *EastEnders* was finished! Never mind *EastEnders*, I was about ready to burst with excitement! I made sure that my mother knew what was happening, and Michelle's mother was already with us, so we all travelled to hospital together. But only after *EastEnders*!

I couldn't believe that it was finally happening. We were going to have a baby! I think there was a small part of me that was scared of what was to come, but, mostly, I was just so happy. I felt as if this was the beginning of the rest of our lives.

But if life (and *EastEnders*) teaches us anything, it's that things don't often work out the way you've planned ...

CHAPTER 5

The hospital was only about two miles away, and we got there without a hitch. They didn't think there was any doubt that Michelle was close, so they ushered us straight through to the ward, and we had the place to ourselves.

I was so excited, but the nerves were really creeping in. I didn't know what to expect. I tried to remember what I had seen in the antenatal classes, but my brain went blank. When the nurse came in, she told Michelle to put on a gown and then checked how far the baby had moved.

We were all hoping for a quick birth; Michelle's sister had been in and out in a few hours. But the nurse told us we were going to have to wait: Michelle had started labour, but the baby wasn't ready to be born yet. I should have known – Michelle has always been late for everything, and I guess my son was going to live up to his mother's habits.

We talked for a bit and listened to cheesy love songs on the radio. Even now, when I hear certain songs, it brings back the memory of that night as we waited for our son to be born.

I went to get us all a cup of tea, and phoned my friends to keep them up to date. And that's when I saw him ... an old friend of mine was walking unsteadily down the corridor towards me. He looked really unwell. I told him that I was there for my baby's birth, and he wished me good luck with it.

We'd been friends a long time. Like me, he had a reputation for doing crazy things. I remember once, he was challenged to go into a pub naked, and order a pint. He did it without a second thought. Much like me, he had a reputation as a drinker. It was well deserved. But his body couldn't take it any more. He was in hospital because he'd been drinking himself into an early grave. His body was giving up on him.

That was the last time I saw him. That night – and that meeting – still bring up so many emotions. I know that when I went back up to Michelle, I was starting to feel even more anxious. I didn't know anything about what was happening. I sipped on my tea to try to calm myself down, but I was still panicking a little. I needed things to happen, and they weren't. Being patient has never been one of my best qualities, so I couldn't handle just sitting there.

My mum showed up, and was so excited for the arrival of her grandchild. The two experienced mums (and now grans-to-be) knew there was no point stressing; we just had to sit back and wait for things to happen. It was great to have their support. Another two hours passed, and the nurse told us we'd need to wait another couple of hours. Ten hours later, we were still waiting. Eventually they moved us to another room, and tried to make Michelle as comfortable as they could.

I asked the nurse what was happening, but she never explained anything. She just told us everything was fine, and we had to wait. I felt useless. I wanted to support Michelle, but there was nothing for me to do. No money for me to earn, no food for me to buy, nothing practical I could offer. I felt like a bystander. Other families who had come in after us were wheeled out. They all seemed to be getting on with it, and I couldn't help but question why it wasn't happening for us.

Still we waited. Around the 15-hour mark, I was so exhausted, so emotionally drained, that I just wanted to sleep. I didn't want to be selfish though. Michelle was really uncomfortable now, so I just kept walking around and talking. I can't even remember what I was saying, but I knew I had to stay awake. I couldn't understand why it was taking so long. It wasn't supposed to be like this, was it? Something was wrong. I was convinced of it. I didn't say anything out loud, but I couldn't stop that niggling doubt from growing in my heart.

It had never occurred to me before that day that someone could be in labour for so long. I had only heard of people who were in and out before dinnertime! But it was coming close to 18 hours, and my face felt like it was going to explode with the stress of waiting.

Nearly a full day after we'd arrived, three doctors came in to tell us that they needed to carry out an emergency caesarean section. There were no reassuring words, or comfort; it was all so matter-of-fact. They looked how I felt: unhappy, stressed, worried. I was looking to them for reassurance, but they didn't have any to give me.

I started to feel dizzy and I was scared that I was going to faint. I didn't realise it at the time, but I was having a panic attack. It was awful. The midwife could see that I was struggling and started to help me – but that just made me feel worse. I didn't want them taking attention away from Michelle. In the end, I think the only thing stopping me from passing out was the fact that it would be so embarrassing. I didn't want to be one of those funny stories: the man who passed out while his wife gave birth!

But I just felt so confused. And I felt robbed of what I had imagined was going to happen. I had dreamt up something in my head, and the reality wasn't anything like that. I wanted to cut the cord, I wanted to hold onto my wife's hand as she pushed, I wanted the whole experience. The experience my dad had never had. But now I was going to get something different, something that I had never even heard of – and I simply didn't know how to deal with any of it.

As I looked at Michelle, I knew that she was feeling a lot of the same things as me. My heart was racing, and I sensed that something was very wrong. I didn't know what was going to happen. I was terrified, for Michelle and for my baby.

I felt so weak standing there, next to Michelle, not knowing what to do. One of the doctors handed me a bag to breathe in. I hated feeling out of control, and, more than that, I hated feeling like I was letting Michelle down. In my mind, I had always been Michelle's protector. I felt secure in that role. But at that moment, I felt so weak.

When they took Michelle into the delivery theatre, she was exhausted. I was in complete and utter admiration of her for the way she handled the situation. I just wanted this ordeal to be over for her. I wanted us to be that happy couple, stepping out of hospital into a bright new day, our baby tucked up safely in his carry-cot. But then I saw the instruments they'd be using to cut Michelle open.

A C-section is a major surgical operation, but I didn't know what it involved. Perhaps it was because they didn't explain what they were actually going to do, or maybe it was just because I was so very tired, but I couldn't catch my breath. I was sweating and my heart began to race so fast that I thought it might stop.

That's when all of my fears grew into one terrifying image: my wife and child were going to die.

Somehow, I stayed on my feet. I don't really remember much of what happened next. But when our son – when our beautiful baby, Ethan – was safely born on 1st December 2004 at 2.16pm, after more than 20 hours in labour and a 30-minute operation, the relief washed over me. I had genuinely thought Michelle and my baby were going to die.

Now that it was finally over, I hoped that we could put this nightmare behind us. Then I heard him cry – he had arrived into the world with a good set of lungs – and I remember feeling tingles all over my body and the hairs on the back of my neck standing on end.

After you've been waiting so long for your own flesh and blood to arrive, there's an intense moment when they hand your baby to you for the first time. That's when they say you experience an amazing feeling of intimacy and closeness. But the devastating truth is I didn't experience any of that. After all of the anguish we had suffered, there was no happiness; I just felt cheated and bitter. The baby in my hands was something that I had been waiting all this time for, but now he was here, I couldn't bring myself to feel anything for him.

CHAPTER 6

I couldn't get past what I'd experienced. Seeing the person you love going through something so traumatic had a lasting impact on me. I kept playing it back in my mind – the horror of seeing my wife being cut open, of Ethan being taken out of her ... the blood.

Years later, I would find out about traumatic experiences in the labour ward, but back then, I didn't know anything about it. All I knew was that I had been deeply affected by what I had seen. Still, to this day, the thought of seeing my wife with a baby-size bump under her clothes makes me shiver with dread. I couldn't handle the idea of walking into a labour room and going through it again. I still can't.

We had made the decision to have children so quickly. It had been the easiest decision in the world. Now, we made the decision not to have any more children. Just as easily. Just as quickly. Neither one of us wanted to go through that ordeal again. My visions of the future shifted. Now there would only be one little Williams.

For weeks after the birth, I would see the knives from the tray next to Michelle whenever I closed my eyes. I could just imagine the way they would slice into her body, the blood, the pain of it all. I could see it, hear it, smell it all so clearly in my head.

I had been waiting for that day for so long, but when it came, I hated it.

I had hated seeing Michelle looking so weak and small and alone as she lay there. And I had hated feeling so helpless, so useless. I was nothing.

I knew nothing would ever be the same again. Michelle and I were changed by the experience – and now, we had to adjust to our new lives as parents ...

The first few hours after the birth brought a mix of emotions. When I looked down at Ethan, holding him in my arms, I didn't feel anything but relief that it was over. Relief that he was safe. Relief that no one had died. I had wanted to feel the joy of holding my son in my arms for the first time. But it was only relief.

As I looked across to Michelle, who was lying in the bed watching us, I told her I was glad that he didn't have my big, bony, bent nose. She laughed, and then told me to check his ears, which were small, unlike mine. We both breathed a sigh of relief at that one; I couldn't imagine a baby with my nose or my ears.

As some of the immediate anxiety drained away, I remember thanking the doctors who had done their work so well. I held my hand out to them, thanking them in the only way I knew how. I was still feeling angry, but I knew that they had done something amazing. And I wanted them to understand what they meant to me, for what they had done for my family.

When Michelle was given Ethan, she gently touched his face, as though she didn't quite understand what she was holding, and then placed him close to her skin. She seemed quiet, as though she still didn't quite know how to process everything she had been through. When we went back to the ward, I told her I wanted to go into town, to ring people and tell them our news.

'Please, don't go,' she said, simply.

She didn't say why, but I knew she needed me there with her. By her side. Something didn't feel right; as if something had changed inside her. At the time, I assumed that she was emotionally and physically exhausted from the birth. I thought that this was the norm for new mums. So I stayed until the nurses told me to go and get some rest.

As I left the ward, the only thing I could think about was having a glass of wine and a few lagers. I told myself it was to toast the arrival of my son. But deep down I knew I needed the alcohol to help me feel numb. I could still remember everything I had seen, and I wanted to push the images out of my head. I couldn't even begin to imagine what it had been like for Michelle to go through all of that.

I couldn't focus on it any more, so I headed straight to the local shop and bought myself a few drinks on the way home.

As I put the key in the door, our house seemed so lonely and empty and dark. The second I stepped in, I knew that I couldn't stay there. I went back outside and saw the lights were on in our neighbours' house. I knocked at the door and told them the news.

To my relief, they invited me in and we had a few drinks. I kept talking about how everything had gone with the birth. I had been in their house before for drinks, but this time, I felt like a different person. I was a father now, and that meant something. After I left their house to get some sleep, I kept thinking about my new responsibilities as a dad …

I got some sleep, but it was a restless night, and I still felt tired when I woke up. It was December, and the house was so cold, as well as empty. Everything felt so dream-like. Everything felt strangely significant, like I was doing it for the first time as a father.

I couldn't wait to get back to the hospital. All that mattered now was making sure they were alright. But as I approached the ward, I could see Michelle sitting on a chair, her hands firmly gripping the sides, and staring straight ahead. Ethan was asleep, his tiny hands curled into fists. When she saw me, she told me she hadn't had any sleep, as one of the other women on the ward had been snoring throughout the night. She told me she wanted to come home with me, to her own bed. But the nurses told her she had to stay in hospital and rest for three days after her C-section.

Rest?!

My wife was in a room filled with crying babies and mothers snoring. How was she meant to get any rest here? I thought they'd put her into a private room. After all, most of the other mothers in the room had had normal births. Michelle hadn't, and she'd been awake for at least 48 hours.

We talked while she checked on Ethan, but it was an effort for her. She seemed so pale and broken, not like my Michelle. Of course she was tired. She'd had a traumatic experience and she was exhausted. I didn't think anything else was wrong ...

The nurse asked me if I wanted to bathe Ethan. I was a little nervous, but she showed me what to do, and even offered to capture the moment. I still have that photo of us together like that, me holding Ethan, fear and the first stirrings of love etched on my face! I couldn't quite feel the full force of love yet, but deep down, I think I knew that this boy was going to become the most important person in our lives. I washed and powdered him, and put his nappy on – the first of countless nappies to come.

After visiting time was over, Michelle asked if I was going to come back in for the night. She seemed so lost and needy, it just wasn't like her. She had always been so strong and confident. I don't think anything had ever beaten her before, but this was different. I wanted to stay, but the nurses told me it would be better for us both if I went home. Looking back now, I wonder what might have happened if I hadn't given in, if I had stayed with her that night.

After having heard that he'd finally arrived, friends and family started to visit Ethan that day. I could see that this was hard for Michelle. She kept trying to put on a brave face, but she looked like she was crying inside. I guess everybody expects that you should be dancing around from sheer happiness when you've had a baby, but that's not true for everyone, or even for most people. The experience can be utterly exhausting – both mentally and physically. And the more you try to hide your real feelings, the harder it can be.

I knew that I wasn't experiencing the sorts of feelings that people said I would be. I love Ethan more than life itself, and he comes before anyone else. But when he was born, I didn't have the overwhelming surge of feelings that other people said they had. He was a stranger to me, just a small baby that I couldn't understand. I grew to love him as the days and weeks and months went on, just like you do when you fall in love with anyone. But in those early days, it was hard. I don't know if it was because the birth had gone so wrong, but I was starting to doubt myself as a father. Was I feeling this way because of the C-section? Was it connected to the panic attacks I had before the birth? Was it just me being stupid, and over-thinking every little thing I was doing?

When I think of the whole birth and hospital experience, it had such a major impact on the rest of our lives in so many different ways. The hospital was completely excellent, and the staff did exactly what was required of them. But I just wish that someone had sat me down right then and there and told me that what I was feeling was completely normal. I needed to know that many, many people experience the beginnings of parenthood like this. I needed to know that there was nothing wrong with me. But no one ever did talk to me. No one ever answered my questions.

Antenatal classes are supposed to prepare you for what happens, but after that, you're on your own. Having a baby is such a profoundly big change in people's lives; I couldn't understand how there wasn't more support available to us. It felt as if we'd been cheated out of our experience of childbirth.

Perhaps if I had understood more about the C-section, if I had been told that it was something that might happen, or if I had been told about all the conflicting emotions I might have felt after

Ethan was born, then maybe things would have been different. But I'll never know. That wasn't the hand I was dealt.

I have since found out that a "doula" can act as a go-between for the mothers and nurses, but we were never offered that kind of support. Or perhaps it just wasn't available at the time. Either way, we were entirely on our own.

When I left the hospital that second night, I decided I was going to stay at my mother's house. I didn't fancy going home to an empty house again. I slept well and the next morning, I went home to make the house ready for Ethan and Michelle to come home to. In between jobs, I'd phone the ward to check on Ethan and Michelle. They said they were both doing fine.

But when I went back to the hospital, I found Michelle staring blankly across the ward again. She didn't seem fine to me at all. It certainly didn't feel like the happiest time in our lives.

I started asking myself: wasn't this everything that we'd wanted? Didn't Michelle want this? Didn't she want to be a mother? Or, was it just me?

I sat beside her and asked what was wrong. I wanted to try to find something – anything – I could do to help. I don't know what I expected her to say, but when she said she felt frightened and scared, I was surprised. I didn't understand what was left to be scared of; the birth had been terrible, but it was over now. Surely, this was the start of the best times of our lives?

I didn't know what to think. I wondered if there was something she wasn't telling me. When I was talking to her, she seemed mostly fine, but she never wanted me to leave her side. She looked completely terrified if I left the ward for a few minutes. I knew that Ethan was safe and well, and that was one reassurance, but Michelle wasn't the same person who had entered the hospital with me all those days ago.

Where was my Michelle?

CHAPTER 7

I was taking my new family home.

Michelle was quiet. She just wanted to get home and try to catch up on some sleep. We settled Ethan into the car seat for the first time, and quietly drove home. Neither one of us was able to speak to the other.

Maybe it would be better when we got home?

I remember walking into our little two-bedroom house and suddenly thinking how much we were going to need a bigger house to fit the clothes, the pram, the cot, the baby bath, all the other gear needed by a new family. As I closed the door behind me, it felt weird. It was as though the house had suddenly shrunk before my eyes.

We now had the responsibility of looking after a baby human 24 / 7. Now that's something they definitely hadn't taught me in school. When there's a tiny new somebody in the house, things change, and they change fast.

The house suddenly went from the quiet and empty place it had been a few days ago to a place full of noise, with absolutely no room. It felt as though our entire lives had been hijacked.

I could see from the moment that we started to live together as a family of three that Michelle wasn't right. She seemed to do everything half-heartedly, as though she didn't really care about anything. She was very quiet, just as she had been in hospital. She didn't even seem like she was on the same planet as the rest of us. But I kept putting it all down to exhaustion. I didn't think there was anything else going on.

I kept asking if there was anything I could do, but she didn't respond in her normal way. It was her body language that scared me most: her shoulders were lowered, her back was hunched, her lips were constantly drooped down. It was as though someone had cut the strings from her body, and she looked like she was close to collapsing.

Michelle wasn't interested in having visitors at home either. It seemed so overwhelming for her. I could see that she just wanted them to go away and leave her completely alone. Every time someone came into the house, she looked uncomfortable. Her voice was low and quiet, her answers to questions were quick and to the point. Sometimes, our visitors would pick up on it and leave; other times, they would stay, and all the while Michelle was shrinking away from them, becoming more and more withdrawn.

Those first few months were awful for sleep. I was used to going out like a light, but Michelle was always tossing and turning. I wouldn't get to sleep unless I knew she was asleep too, but she just couldn't, no matter how much she tried.

Sometimes, she would shake me awake in the middle of the night because she was feeling scared, and would ask me all sorts of questions. I never knew what to do and it felt as though I was letting her down, as if she wanted something from me that I couldn't give her. It started to seem as if Michelle was getting paranoid, like she doubted everything that I told her. And as the days went by, she became more and more withdrawn. She wasn't eating enough, she spent longer in bed during the day, and didn't sleep at night. She never left the house I wish I knew then what I know now, but I didn't realise just how big an impact the birth had had on her.

After about a week of this, we were up at my mum's when the health visitor came around to see us for a check-up. (That's a routine service for all new mums and babies.) After spending some time with us, she told us she was very concerned. This was the first time I had ever heard anyone say the words "postnatal depression" (PND).

Even though I knew the health visitor must be right, I still couldn't quite get my head around it. Why would Michelle be depressed? We had a beautiful baby, a lovely house, good jobs, and great holidays. How could she want anything more?

But the health visitor was convinced. All the signs were there, so she had to put us in touch with the mental health team. Mental health team? How could this be happening? I fought with the words in my head. I didn't know who to blame – and I needed to blame someone. Was it my fault? Didn't she want us to be a family ... or was it me she didn't want? I had so many questions racing through me, questions that I couldn't ask out loud.

When Gail from the mental health team rang later, she was straight, firm, and very understanding of what we were going through. She told me that depression wasn't something that Michelle could just stop feeling. It wouldn't be quite as easy as that, no matter how much we wanted it to be. She told us she'd be there to help Michelle through this, and to help me help her.

Gail made an appointment to visit Michelle the following day so they could have a face-to-face chat. It was a relief to hear that; it meant that someone was coming who'd know what to do with Michelle. Help was on the way.

I know that people think depression is something you can snap out of. They believe, like I did, that it's the same thing as being in a low mood the day after drinking, or not wanting to go to work on a Monday morning. I know as well as anyone that you can just about force yourself into work with a hangover, but getting out of depression just isn't that easy. Mental illness is never that straightforward.

Gail came back to speak to Michelle again the next day, but I wasn't allowed to be there. I now see that it was important for it to happen the way it did, but at the time, that was tough to take.

Gail, or another lovely lady called Sue, were there whenever Michelle needed them, which was often. They made sure she had help looking after Ethan any time she felt like she was struggling. As the days went by, Michelle became worse and worse, despite the help, so my mum looked after Ethan while I took Michelle out shopping. She needed to get out of the house – have a change of scene. We'd been saving so hard, so I told her to go mad and buy whatever she wanted. She just looked at me and said, 'It doesn't matter. It won't change how I feel inside.' Her voice was lifeless, there was no feeling or emotion there. It felt like she was becoming someone else. The Michelle I knew was just fading away before my eyes, and there was nothing that I could do about it.

It felt like my best friend had left me, and all that was left was this baby that I had no idea how to care for.

I felt so alone. More alone than I had ever felt in my life.

I began to doubt myself as a new father. I felt like I must be the only man, the only new father, who had ever gone through this. After all, if it happened to anyone else, wouldn't someone have told me about it?

It's not as if I'd thought everything was going to be fine when Ethan came around – I knew it wouldn't be easy – but I had never imagined things were going to be this bad. I'd hoped that if we'd run into problems we'd have worked through them together. Not like this, not separate and alone.

I remember Michelle didn't want me to tell anyone about her illness, which made me feel even more alone. She said that people might think badly of her, or call her a bad mother, as though she had something missing from her. I knew that this couldn't be further from the truth; even when she was in her deepest depressions, she was still the most loving person I had ever known. She was still a great mother, despite being so ill. But still I had to stay quiet.

So I set about my new routine, trapped in loneliness. And I struggled. With dirty nappies and middle-of-the-night feedings, it felt like a mountain to climb. For every step forwards, there were three steps back.

There were good things, memories I'll cherish, like when Ethan got his first tooth, or when he said his first word, or when he crawled for the first time. But the day-to-day caring for a baby began to take its toll on me.

Our house no longer felt like a home. It wasn't the same open place for people to pop in and visit, it had turned into a hiding place. Michelle would curl up on a sofa, or in bed, and she would cut herself off from everyone. I began to feel isolated. I couldn't go out, I couldn't invite anyone around, and I couldn't be with Michelle.

We didn't know how long Michelle was going to be like this – weeks? Months? Years? We asked the nurses when we could expect her to move past it, but there was no way they could answer that. They told us that discovering it quickly was a positive, as some women never sought or received any help, and had to live their lives trapped in the smog with no way out.

We were lucky. We had the support of our families and friends. And I was so thankful for the help we got from the health visitor and the nurses. If we hadn't been able to rely on them whenever Michelle felt ill, I don't know what we would have done.

But in spite of all their help, there was still worse to come ...

CHAPTER 8

Michelle and I tried to go with the flow, and to just accept what came our way. But as the Christmas holidays approached, we felt the pressure more and more, knowing that we would be expected to join in the festivities. For others, it was still the most wonderful time of the year, but for us, it wasn't the same. Our home had become Michelle's hiding place from the rest of the world. And now, it was mine too. Sometimes, we didn't feel like we wanted to put a brave face on. Sometimes, it was great to just hear the door lock behind us as we walked in, safe in our own little world. Sometimes, it was nice to just be on our own.

We tried to make the best of things in our own little world. But sometimes, it was all too much to cope with. Just trying to get Ethan ready felt like a Herculean task, and it would take us an hour just to walk around the corner. If Michelle was having a bad day, I would have to try to get her out of bed too, and everything just took even longer. It was, in a sense, like looking after two children, trying to get both of them up and out of the house.

Like everyone else, I've had ups and downs in my life, but I had never experienced anything like this before. Coming home to Michelle in the old days had been like paradise; now, it was like my own special version of hell.

Sometimes, I would come into the bedroom and see Michelle hiding under the duvet, curled up in a ball. I would lift the duvet, and find her crying inconsolably. When I asked her what was wrong, she couldn't tell me. So I'd just sit there with her, waiting for her to come to, waiting for something to get better. But there were never any easy answers. Just more problems. Our lives were stuck. We were trapped.

That young Mark meeting Michelle in the nightclub would never in a million years have thought his life would turn out like this.

I was desperate. Sometimes, I would just stand by our window and see the cross on the local chapel, and I would pray to God that it would all go away.

Whenever I saw people laughing or having fun, I hated it. I hated them. How dare they have such a good time when we were going through so much?

I often cried. I don't feel any shame in saying that. There was a deep sorrow inside me trying to get out. A sense of mourning for what I'd lost. For what we'd thought we were going to get.

I felt in my heart that my life wasn't ever going to be good again. It was just too far gone. A part of me still hoped that perhaps we could turn things around, perhaps we could still, somehow, claw back the life we had imagined for ourselves. But every time I looked in Michelle's eyes, I felt as if we were lost. We had given up. This was our life now. And there was no coming back from it.

As Christmas came crawling towards us, we put up the tree and decorated it, just as if everything was normal. But we were just pretending. Pretending was all we had left. I had always loved this time of year, and it had always meant so much to me, but it felt different this time. I didn't know how to be a good father. Or a good husband. I didn't know how to be happy any more.

I hated that Christmas. I can still remember how happy everyone else seemed to be, which just made it worse. For everyone else there were huge smiles, big stomachs, and love and warmth. But there was none of that inside me. I hated my life.

Helpless. Useless. Worthless.

I hadn't gone back to work. I couldn't face it. The money we'd set aside was long gone, and the debts were mounting. It seemed as if I was slowly losing touch with reality. I felt like nothing. I didn't care about anything. I just wanted to escape.

Every day was getting worse. Mentally. Physically. Financially. I wanted to move on, but there was nowhere to go.

With no other income coming into the house, I had to see if there was any more support out there for Michelle, beyond the nurses and the health visitor. But though it seemed that everyone was aware of postnatal depression, there wasn't much in the way of practical support available for families in need. Today, thankfully, there are specialist services for postnatal mental health, but back in 2005, there were hardly any resources for mothers, fathers and couples in need.

During Christmas, as if things weren't bad enough, we found out that a very close friend of ours had passed away. I had only seen this friend a few weeks ago in the hospital, while I was waiting for Ethan to be born. I could hardly believe it. He was only a few years older than me. And I couldn't help but wonder what might have changed if he had been given the help that he needed. He was only 36 when he died, barely half a life.

On the day of the funeral, Michelle stayed with her sister so that I could forget about things at home. The last thing I wanted was to be reminded of everything else that was going on, and it also meant that I could go out for a few drinks in the afternoon, which I was looking forward to.

I know that drink can be like a siren call when you're experiencing feelings of despair or depression, and I drank what felt like a barrel or more that day. It helped me to forget some of the sadness, just for a moment or two. And it felt good to be around friends again, even under the sad circumstances. I felt almost normal for once. I was just Mark. Not Mark the father, not Mark the depressed husband. Just Mark.

As I sat there in the pub, I cast a glance over everyone else. And I started to wonder how many of them were depressed, just like I was. I looked at each of my friends in turn. How many of them could even begin to guess the truth of what was happening behind my closed doors? How many of them would ever imagine what we were going through?

I couldn't say anything though. Here we were, mourning our friend, but even then, the normal rules applied. It wasn't the time or the place to talk about our feelings. It never was. I started to feel uneasy, as if the depression might show through in my face. I didn't want them to find out, and if they did, I didn't want them to find out this way. It sounds stupid looking back now, but I didn't want to show any weakness. As a man, I felt like I shouldn't even know how that felt. But I did. I knew all too well how it felt to be made powerless and paralysed by depression – and I hated it.

The next few days were a total nightmare. I returned home with a huge hangover, and had to look after both Michelle and Ethan. I knew things were getting worse when Michelle said she wanted her mother to move in with us to help her look after Ethan.

Over the next few days, Michelle's mood was all over the place, so we asked for more help. The medication she was on wasn't working; it made her uneasy and edgy. And then there were the sleeping tablets that she had to take. She said that her mind felt as though it was on overload; it was constantly running, but she found it hard to concentrate on anything. Watching a film or reading a book was out of the question; she just couldn't pay attention for that long.

We knew it could take two or three weeks for the effects of the new medication to kick in. That was hard on Michelle who was so desperately tired and still finding it hard to sleep. So we moved into my parents' house for a while; it made her feel safe. We sat on my bed, in the room where I had grown up, and looked out of the window together. We couldn't believe how little time had passed; just four weeks since Ethan's birth, and yet it had felt like a lifetime.

With 2004 coming to an end, we hoped that New Year might bring better days.

We had always celebrated New Year's Eve, and we had already made our plans before Ethan had been born. He spent the night with our family, while Michelle and I went to our neighbours' house-party with Michelle's sister and her partner. Our neighbours were very welcoming and didn't have a clue what was happening in our lives. It was great to let our hair down and just have a good time.

But more than that, it was nice to see Michelle that night. It was as though she was back from the dead, alive and happy again. She didn't drink because of her medication, but the change in her made it feel as if she had downed the same amount as I had. To look at her, you would never have known she was going through the worst experience of her life. She looked like someone who didn't have a care in the world, someone who was enjoying all that life had to give. It gave me hope, watching her that night, and I assumed that this might be it. This might be the turning point. We had been through the war, and now we were coming to the end of it. As the party wound down, I wasn't sure what to expect, but I was optimistic about the morning ...

Unfortunately, as much as I hoped it would be, this wasn't the end of it. Before the new year was a few hours old, the nightmare returned. It was as if it had never gone away. I can't tell you how hard it was to experience that. I had got my Michelle back, but only for a single night. I had allowed myself to believe that our lives would go back to normal. But Michelle wasn't okay. She was only pretending to be.

And that was even worse. I was the only person who knew the truth. As far as everyone else was concerned, we were fine. They saw a happy young couple with a baby, but they didn't see what happened when we let our guard down.

It was like when people asked me what it was like at the birth. And I'd usually tell them all the right things, all the things I knew they wanted to hear. They were the same things that I had wanted to hear when I talked to mums and dads before Ethan arrived.

But sometimes, if I knew they really wanted to hear the honest truth, I'd tell them that I'd felt cheated. I'd tell them that we'd been expecting a normal birth, and that I'd imagined holding Michelle's hand, then cutting the cord, and holding my baby. I'd tell them that I'd been looking forward to seeing one of life's miracles happen before my eyes, and that it never happened.

Men have their own stories to tell. Of the exhilaration and the excitement, and the tiredness and the happiness. Some say they felt high on it all. And I listen to their stories, wondering why I had never got to experience any of that. Wondering where my slice of the pie was.

Michelle's illness was quickly getting worse, and I began to fear for her safety. I wanted her back. I would have given everything I had to get her back to the way she was before Ethan was born.

But, bad as it was, I didn't think it could get any worse, until the day I had to call Gail and her team, and tell them to take Michelle to the hospital.

We were coming back from her mother's house in Bristol when she suddenly felt like she couldn't cope any more. She said she was scared, terrified to her bones. As we drove on the motorway, she said she didn't care if we crashed, because at least Ethan would be taken care of by other people. She said that ultimately, he would be better off if that happened. She just wanted the constant and agonising pain within her to stop.

To this day, whenever I see the empty eyes of people going through PND, I am reminded of the living hell she endured.

It was so awful to know that she was so lost. Michelle was such a deeply loving person with so very much to give. But in that moment, it felt like she really was gone forever. I feared I was never going to get back my wife, my best friend in the entire world.

There was no one I could turn to. I couldn't tell my friends, because Michelle still wanted to keep it a secret. And I couldn't tell my family about the way I was feeling, because they needed to focus on Michelle.

So I just carried on carrying on.

Ten signs that you might be suffering from postnatal depression:

1. You may feel an increased sensitivity to anger, which can lead to increased conflicts with those around you

2. You might become easily frustrated or irritated by small things

3. You may turn to alcohol, or other substances, far more than usual, using them to make yourself feel better

4. You might find yourself losing or gaining a significant amount of weight

5. You might become more impulsive than usual

6. You may begin to suffer from physical problems, such as headaches, body aches / pain, and digestive problems

7. You may begin to lose your ability to concentrate much on tasks

8. You may begin to lose interest in your work, hobbies, and personal interests

9. You might start to feel conflicted between what you feel a man should be and what you currently are

10. You may start to think of suicide or death

CHAPTER 9

January brought cold, dark days and nights, and the comedown after Christmas was long and bitter. I knew that I needed to get back to work; I wasn't earning anything sitting at home! We were hitting the credit cards hard, and the post-Christmas bills were starting to flood in. I wasn't entitled to any state benefits while I was off either, so money was getting really tight.

It all came to a head one evening at the end of January. It started off as normal – well, normal for what we were currently going through. As we were sat there watching TV, Ethan started crying and wouldn't stop. I didn't know it at the time, but this was going to be the longest night of my life. Ethan carried on crying as we changed his nappy ... and as we tried to feed him ... and as we tried to comfort him. In desperation, we put him back to bed and hoped he'd quieten down. He didn't. We just couldn't understand what was wrong. It was horrible. And then Michelle just edged towards the stairs, turned to me, and with no emotion in her voice told me she was off to bed. I watched her leave, and she didn't look back once.

Ethan hadn't paused for air. If you've ever spent a few minutes with a distressed baby, you'll know just how hard that is. It was too late to phone anyone, and as I stood there, feeling more alone and more stressed than I had ever felt in my life, all the pent-up pressure and stress hit me all at once. Ethan kept crying and crying and crying, and I didn't know what I was doing. I was pacing back and forth, my heart racing, and then I just collapsed on the sofa with my head in my hands.

I was shaking now. I went into the bedroom and told Michelle to get up and help me. She reacted by hiding under the sheets and ignoring me. I even thought about dragging her from the bed. I left her there and went into Ethan's, who hadn't stopped crying for a second. I went to change him again, thinking this might help, but it didn't. In fact, he ended up peeing all over me. It went everywhere – all over the cot, the sheets, his clothes. The stress rose again and a headache to go with it. I shouted at him, 'Why are you crying?!' I felt so angry, it was like I was seeing red.

I left him then, to compose myself before I ended up doing something I would regret. I gave it a few minutes, and then went back in, picked him up and cuddled him. But still he cried. I never liked doing it, but I gave him some medicine to try to settle him. I couldn't bear to think about another day like this. I was getting desperate.

I bundled Ethan into the car and went to my parents for help. I hated running to them for help, but didn't have any choice. I was at the lowest point now: I couldn't look after my own wife and child. I could barely look my parents in the eyes as they let us in. I had woken them up in the middle of the night, and I was on the verge of collapse.

Eventually, they managed to calm him down and we all got some fitful sleep. The next morning, I took Ethan home, and called Michelle's mother, Janet. I told her that Michelle needed her help. But because she lived and worked in Bristol, she couldn't just move, and she couldn't just give up her job; it wasn't as simple as that.

Michelle was getting more and more agitated as we talked, and then grabbed the phone from me. She shouted down the phone that she needed her mother. What choice did she have? After talking for a few minutes, Janet agreed to come and stay with us.

I will never forget how grateful I felt. She was there for us when we really needed her, and that meant more to us than anything. She helped so much with Ethan, which meant that I was free to take a few minutes to unwind with a walk, or a quick trip to the pub.

My drinking was getting a little bit out of control. I had managed to keep it under tight control when Michelle was pregnant, when life was full of optimism. But as soon as the stress had started building up, I had felt all the same impulses to drink myself better. It was becoming almost impossible not to drink when things felt so bad. The problem was, because I had made myself such a hardened drinker, my tolerance levels had increased. To get to that magical place where I didn't remember anything, I had to drink more and more.

If I'd been able to, I'd have drunk myself into a stupor every day. The only thing that stopped me was knowing that Michelle and Ethan were worth any hardship. Even in my darkest days, I still hung onto that. I still believed it.

But when I did have a chance to go out with my mates, we really went for it. We went well beyond drunk and into totally smashed territory. I would get really moody and miserable after I had drunk a few and acquired the nickname 'Five Pints' because of it. I had never been like that before. I had always been a happy drunk, always ready to do anything, always the life and soul of any party. But I had lost all of that. Now I was a horrible dark person after only a few pints. The morning after was worse. That's when the paranoia set in. I would see people who had been in the pub or nightclub from the night before, and I would wonder if I had done something to upset them in some way. It was hard not to think like that. I was always so convinced that I had done something stupid in my drunken stupor. I started phoning my friends to check up on 'the other Mark' to see if I'd done anything the night before. They would always tell me nothing had happened, but I didn't even know if I could trust them any more. I was beginning to get bad, just as bad as I'd been in my youth. Except this time, I was drinking to get away from something. Some days, I would make myself so bad that I felt like running away and disconnecting from the real world.

I remember trying to start fights with doormen. I wouldn't have had any chance of beating them up, but maybe I just wanted to hurt myself and take away the feelings I was getting in my head. I couldn't stop my mind from racing, and feeling physical pain felt like the only way I could do it. On one occasion I punched the wooden frame of the sofa, which was totally out of character. I ended up in the hospital with a broken hand and a sling, which obviously made it harder to help with Ethan.

There was no fun. No laughter. No partying. Now, the alcohol only had one use: to help me forget my worries for a while. It was only ever a temporary fix. The day after, when the hangover hit and the crying started and the reality kicked in, it felt a hundred times worse. So I'd want to drink that night too, and the night after, and the night after. I couldn't stop it. My weaknesses were controlling me. My self-control was gone. One drink only ever led to another, and another – as many as I needed to make me forget.

On some level, I knew that I had to stop, or at least cut it down. It had been a long time since I'd done anything to look after myself. So I thought I'd give the gym a go. It seemed like a good way to take out some aggression and make myself feel a bit less dead inside.

It was like drinking. Once I started, I found it hard to stop, and I went to the gym as often as I could. I had my addictive personality to thank for that. But that addictive nature worked in other ways too. Facing another dry evening at home, and Michelle's depression was really bad, I found comfort in food: chocolate, crisps, sweets ... All the junk food I could lay my hands on. I'd always been a big eater, and this didn't help me feel any better about myself. Going to the gym just helped me justify eating more.

I still felt like I was chasing a dream of the life I wanted, one that was still hanging in front of me, but being pulled away every time I got close. Setback followed setback. Michelle's tablets had to be changed again; they just weren't working. The most frustrating part was waiting to see if the new tablets would make any difference – we had to wait yet another three to four weeks, hoping that things would improve and then riding the curve of disappointment when nothing changed. I didn't know how we'd cope if the medicine or the dosage just had to be changed again and again. What if they never found the right medication for her? What if she was never fixed?

All of these questions, with answers that I couldn't ever give, were starting to wear on me, drain me, exhaust me.

Janet told us that we really needed to get out and relax one night while she watched Ethan. I guess she must have felt her own pressures about her daughter's illness. I never asked her how she felt, I wished I had, but it must have had a massive effect on her. Depression is not just an isolated feeling – it can affect everyone around you. As for my sisters-in-law, they didn't know the full extent of the troubles we faced, but they were very concerned about Michelle and her slow recovery. Just knowing they were there – and knowing they could help – was a comfort.

Michelle was feeling positive during the day, so we booked a table at a restaurant. Michelle drove so that I could have a few drinks. It was just like it had been before. Even better than before. Again, I felt like I had my wife back. She even told me how great she was feeling, and said that she'd been telling one or two of her friends about what had happened to her. That really showed me how far she'd come. She had never wanted anyone to know about what she was going through, but now she was telling them. Surely this meant everything was getting better?

Over the next few days, Michelle was so much better than she had been, and it was a wonderful feeling to have her back again. I even started to plan for going back to work, and so did Michelle.

But this horrible illness, which had taken hold of our lives, wasn't finished with us yet. Michelle got ill again, and was soon spending her days in bed. Janet and I tried to encourage her out, but she said she couldn't do it. It felt as if the illness had just taken a break, but now it was back, just as bad as before.

But even though the illness had returned, the truth was, I still had to go back to work. I needed to earn money, and I needed to at least try to get back to normal on my side of things. I needed to escape those four walls.

So I returned to work, and I considered myself lucky because my boss was so understanding of what we were going through. His son was going through his own battle with depression, so he completely understood where I was coming from, and welcomed me back.

Although I was a lone worker, I always had the company of my customers, and I relished the idea of being able to speak to people who didn't know anything about me or what I was going through. But I found that my mindset was completely different when I returned. I was nervous and had lost the confidence that had made me so good at my job before. I felt as if people must be able to see the problems written all over my face.

Every fibre of my being was urging me to run away. And it wasn't long before I walked away after a customer meeting and headed to the nearest pub. I had tried so hard, but I still couldn't cope with it all. I felt myself experiencing the same thoughts as Michelle: I didn't want anyone to know that I was suffering myself. So I sat and drank alone.

I knew that Michelle and Janet were coming to pick me up from work, so I told them to stay home and turned off my phone. I felt like the walls were closing in on me. I felt trapped. There was no way out. One bar led to another, and then a casino. I took in what little money I had, gambled it, and lost it.

Without shame or remorse, I headed back to one last bar and that's when I finally called home to tell people I was safe. My uncle came to pick me up. Of course, he could see that I was drunk, but he could tell that I was upset too. The drive home was silent. The next morning was tense. I felt as if I'd let my family down, and I could tell that they were disappointed with me. But it was only because they couldn't understand why I'd done it. But our community psychiatric nurse (CPN) explained it was a very normal reaction for people in my situation, and that I needed to let off steam. She could tell that I was low, but told me not to be so hard on myself. She said that it was important for me to express myself. And I guess drinking was how I expressed myself – not the best way, of course – but I was good at it!

I was feeling the effects of a deeper, darker depression. And I couldn't do anything to stop it happening. Sometimes, I thought I was alright, and sometimes I wasn't. It felt like I was stuck: I didn't want to move, I didn't want to go anywhere. I wanted to do what Michelle was doing, to just hide away in bed, but I knew I couldn't do that. I had to be the one to support the family, to take care of everyone.

No matter what I tried, I couldn't get back into work. I didn't have the confidence to make sales, and I didn't know if I was ever going to earn a decent wage again. With more hospital appointments, visits from nurses, and phone calls for support, normality seemed to be a long way away for the three of us. I felt like we'd never, ever be a "normal" family.

I wondered if perhaps I just wasn't grown-up enough for all of this. I was then, and still am, very childlike in a lot of ways. And sometimes, I can also act like it. Perhaps I just didn't have the maturity to cope? It felt like I wasn't ready for this responsibility, that we had pulled the trigger too fast, that we should have waited. Or was that just the depression taking hold of me, telling me that everything about myself was wrong?

People started to see a completely different side to me. I became snappy at the smallest of things, and I wanted to be alone at all times, especially when I was drinking. I didn't feel like I could trust myself around other people when I was drunk because I would shout, and fight, and argue. They didn't know what was wrong with me, and I wasn't going to tell them, so I just carried on in the way men do. I wanted desperately to be able to tell them, but how was anyone going to understand what I was going through? How could they?

Weeks went by and everything seemed so flat, so colourless. Everything turned grey. One day, Michelle's mood sank even lower than it had ever been before. I panicked and drove her to the hospital to meet with a specialist. We couldn't go on like this. Something had to be fixed. It was too much for us to handle.

The doctor wanted to admit Michelle, but I wasn't sure. He went to get the paperwork for us to sign, and I pleaded with Michelle to come home. If I had been feeling more secure, I surely wouldn't have stood in her way. But I didn't really know what I was saying any more. I told her that I couldn't survive without her – and I genuinely felt as if I couldn't. I told her Ethan needed his mummy. I talked her around, and Michelle came home with me.

I must have been crazy not to have taken the doctor's advice, not to have even listened to what Michelle herself wanted. But I wasn't thinking straight. I genuinely thought it was the right decision; when we walked around the ward, everyone in there seemed so lifeless and vacant. I didn't want her to spend a single night in there. I would have done anything else to help her, but not this. And then I had this idea that Spain might fix us. The sun and the heat and the people would sort us out. Looking back, I can't believe how naive I was about depression.

Deep down, I know I was scared of being alone with Ethan, scared of not being able to cope, and afraid that I might actually make things worse. Looking back now, I know that I was wrong. I was selfish.

We walked away from the doctor quickly, looking behind us all the way, as though we were going to be caught. It was obviously our decision to make, but I didn't want the doctor to see us and try to change our minds. We went straight home to pack our bags for Spain, but I didn't feel any excitement or happiness; I just felt numb.

We rented a villa with my parents and my maternal grandfather, and put the flights and everything on the credit card. I needed other people around me now, and having my family for support helped take the pressure off me. I felt a little bit human again. It was nice to enjoy the simple things, like breakfast in bed, and just sitting in the sun. My parents were great; they did everything for us and made it feel like a real holiday. It's funny how much I looked for my father's company. I looked forward to having a few drinks with him on the balcony, father to father. My grandfather sat with us too and we watched the planes fly out from Alicante.

We strolled along the beach and went to fancy restaurants in the evenings. Ethan was lapping up all the attention, and didn't stop smiling the entire week. Ethan was really getting into things now, and his personality was starting to show. It was so lovely to watch Michelle playing with him. It was one of the most wonderful things I'd ever seen. I could see the undying love she had for him and I knew she would never do anything to hurt him. It was so sad that she didn't think she could be a good enough mother for him.

Sadly, the week came to an end, as we all knew it would. I would have sold everything I owned to stay in that place. So, we headed back to the airport, and as I held Ethan in my arms, I thought that we would be okay. I dared to believe that this holiday had fixed things. That maybe we were fine.

We boarded the plane, waved goodbye to Spain out of the window, and returned to the grey of the UK. And as we returned, we found that the greyness extended to us too. It wasn't a sudden change, but in the next few days, Michelle's mood fell. We had to go back to the hospital.

I couldn't shake that feeling inside of me, and I wondered again if this was the best thing for Michelle, or for us. But the doctor told us that he only wanted to make Michelle safe. We saw the psychologist again and then the manager of the ward talked to us about the day centre. The day centre didn't seem as bad as the other one we had seen, and it certainly didn't look like the scene from *One Flew Over the Cuckoo's Nest* that I had imagined!

Michelle was booked in to start attending the following week for four hours per day. I could tell that she was feeling a little unsettled at the prospect, so I assured her that she could phone me at any time if she felt like she needed me there.

Finally, Michelle was going to get the help she needed.

CHAPTER 10

Michelle didn't speak much as we headed to the day centre, but she jumped in the car without any hesitation. She didn't speak much as we went in; I think that the fear was starting to loom inside her.

When we got to the ward, everyone seemed so friendly and happy to see us, and I picked up a few leaflets about depression. They told me not to worry; Michelle was in safe hands now. It was oddly like dropping a child off for the first day of school. It was hard to leave, and I felt so lost as she was being led away, like a lost little lamb.

The next few hours went by so slowly. I kept glancing at the clock to see if it was time to go and pick her up and bring her back. I could barely contain myself as I waited. It reminded me of the times I'd spent waiting to go and see Michelle and Ethan on the maternity ward. When it was finally time, I got there as fast as I could.

Michelle seemed okay. She wasn't jumping for joy or anything, but she seemed settled, and told me she was willing to go back for the entire day next time. I couldn't help but feel hopeful when she said that. I was proud of her too. I felt like her recovery was underway, and that she was on the right path to finding herself again. It's strange how a few words, if they're the right words, can change your mind entirely.

For the next few weeks, Michelle continued to go and made some new friends with people from all kinds of backgrounds with various conditions, including post-traumatic stress disorder (PTSD), depression, and trauma.

There wasn't anyone there with PND, but that didn't matter. Michelle never felt judged in any way. She played board games and attended support meetings, she spoke to everyone, she listened, and she learnt.

Being there taught Michelle so much. She started using a mood chart to monitor her feelings, and to record the triggers for her anxiety. That helped her (and me) to begin to pinpoint problems and deal with them more effectively. She started keeping a journal and a daily achievement list to record the things she'd accomplished every day. These tools really helped her to see the changes in her for herself. All she had to do was look back and see how far she'd come.

The people supporting Michelle were amazing. It felt like they'd spend more time with her than they did with their own families. They were so focused on helping her continue on her journey towards recovery. I had been so worried about her going, in case she was hurt or anything, but I saw that it was the safest place for her. And the improvements continued week by week.

That place was a godsend, and we couldn't thank that team of doctors, nurses, and support workers enough. There still need to be more places like this, and there still needs to be so much more funding for the people who do such great work on such small resources.

They say hope is a killer, don't they?

Even with all the help she was getting, and all the progress she was making, the next month was one of the worst times I remember since we had Ethan. Everything had been going so well – or at least that's what I'd thought – but then out of the blue, it fell apart all over again. Michelle started to have suicidal thoughts.

I didn't know at first. The first I knew was when the call came through from the crisis team. I'll never forget the day I found out. It was a Thursday afternoon and I was driving home when I received a phone call saying that Michelle wasn't well, and that she was finding it hard to cope with things. They didn't tell me everything, but it was clear that Michelle was at her lowest ebb. The caller told me to go to the hospital as soon as I could. When I arrived, there were two nurses comforting her. But when she saw me, she was quite still, there was no response from her at all.

I was terrified. I wanted to talk to someone who could just tell me what was going on. I was lost. I kept holding on to my love for Michelle and Ethan. It was all I had left.

The nurse wanted to up her dosage of medication and put a new support plan in place. She was never left alone, with the support worker or Janet there to help her. There were no specialist perinatal mental health services in Wales at that time, but the crisis team made sure she got all the support she needed.

All the while Michelle was in hospital, I looked after Ethan. I found that it was getting easier and easier for me to deal with the daily struggles of having a baby. I could get the bottles ready quicker, and get Ethan ready quicker, and get out of the house quicker. I was starting to feel more and more confident as a father, and was even enjoying the experience. I couldn't ever have imagined feeling like that a few months ago. I loved being around him. I loved him. More and more. Day by day. And that love helped me to cope with the nightmare that Michelle was going through.

Slowly, Michelle started to feel better. We did all the things we had done before, and as the days and weeks went on, her mood stabilised. But even so, I couldn't quite let myself believe that she was completely okay. We had been here before, and I didn't dare let myself hope until it was agreed that Michelle was well enough to go home.

The months went by and Michelle became stronger. The doctors told her to slowly cut her dosage of the medication, and she followed their directions to the letter. After everything she'd been through, she didn't want to take a chance of cutting back too quickly and undoing all the progress she'd made.

Michelle came home, and life returned to some kind of normality. We worked through those days and weeks together, but it was hard. And as Michelle started to get better, I started to feel worse.

I had my wife back, and I was starting to feel like more of a father towards Ethan, but I was still struggling to keep a hold on my depression. I was still snapping at people, still felt angry inside, still felt like I wasn't really me. And I still hadn't told anyone about the way I was feeling. It was all about Michelle and helping her to recover.

I remember coming home to find Janet and Michelle playing board games together. They kept laughing, and although it was a great thing that Michelle was having a good time, I couldn't help feeling angry with them. Every time they laughed, I felt irritated. I went straight to bed to get some rest. I felt so alone.

I suddenly wanted Janet to go home and not come back. I knew that it was good for Michelle to have Janet there, but I couldn't handle it any more. It was my problem, I know that now. But at the time, I was feeling so left out, like I was unimportant, like I had nothing to do. And when I had those feelings, it made me feel guilty, and that made me feel worse. Why did I want someone to leave who had been doing so much to help us? Just because they were laughing!

Deep down, I didn't feel important any longer. I was happy that Michelle was getting back to where she had been before, but I was feeling as though my importance had been taken away from me. I tried to put these feelings away, to the back of my mind, but they stayed there.

I hated feeling like I was angry all the time. I hated being one red flag away from shouting and raving, and arguing and fighting. But it seemed like the only response I had left.

Conversation got more and more strained. I honestly think that if we hadn't been as close to one another as we had been before the illness, we wouldn't still be together today. This illness tested us daily, and at times, I did wonder if we were going to make it through.

Michelle had come so far, and, with her maternity leave coming to an end, she was just starting to think about going back to work. She'd carry on seeing the care team, and she would still have to take things slowly, we all knew that. But she was keen to grab the chance, and prove that she could do it.

We met for lunch in Cardiff on her first day back, to see how the morning had gone. She looked so pale and white, and seemed to not want to make eye contact with me. For the first time in a long time, I found it hard to say anything to her. When she finally looked at me, I waited for her to say something, but she didn't. The moment passed and we carried on eating. We exchanged a few words here and there, but she was so quiet. I wanted to listen to her concerns, and to reassure her, but she didn't give me anything to latch onto.

Years later, I found out that although Michelle continued to go to work, she would go to the local library during her lunchbreak. And cry. Every single day.

After all this time, it still amazes me that she managed to get up every day and go to work, feeling like that. She had so much courage. If I'm honest, I would have run away from that situation, or ended up in the pub, hiding from my feelings.

I was back at work full time too. My boss had told me not to come back until I was good and ready, but I didn't want to let him down, and I didn't want to let Michelle down. I was on commission only by then, so the pressure was on to close every sale. I wanted to hit all my targets, to prove that I was back, to show that I was still good at my job. But with the way things were, I wasn't very good at anything. The old fire was gone, and the easy relationships I'd had with my customers were a thing of the past.

I found that it was getting harder and harder to concentrate. I'd always been forgetful, ever since school, but it was getting worse. I was losing my keys and my cards and my wallet. I would put things down somewhere, then forget where I'd put them, and spend hours trying to find them. It was like my mind was coming apart at the seams. And then I'd get anxious about the likelihood of losing things, because I knew that my family would make some funny remark about me. They quickly learnt not to give me anything to look after, knowing I'd probably lose it within minutes.

Still wrestling with it all, not knowing where to turn, I bumped into an old friend on the way to work one day. For once, my guard slipped, and we just started talking about PND. He told me that his wife had had PND. She hadn't slept and was moody, but according to him, she got over it in a week or two. 'She was strong and just snapped out of it,' he said. I didn't say anything, but I felt like he was wrong. His wife hadn't had PND. Or, at least, she hadn't had it to the same extent that Michelle did. I didn't know it at the time, but he'd been talking about the baby blues that most new mothers experience. That wasn't PND. Not even close.

I wondered why he had told me that. It just made me feel like more of a failure. I'd been so eager to talk to someone who I thought had been through what I'd been through. But instead, he just told me that it was all over, that it had been easy for him, and that his wife was stronger than mine.

Around that time, I bumped into a friend's mother – a nurse I'd known for many years. She had seen us coming out of the ward, and she already suspected some of it. So I hesitantly told her half of my story. I could have told her everything about my experiences and my feelings, but I held back. I don't know why, but I guess part of me still felt like this whole thing was my fault.

It was my fault that Michelle felt the way she did. So I didn't get to tell people about what was going on with me. I didn't deserve that chance to feel better.

I wish I had really talked to my friends about the depression I was feeling. But I couldn't find the words to express myself, and it would have felt like I was somehow going behind Michelle's back. I know my friends wouldn't have judged me, or her, but I really didn't want everyone to think that she was a bad mother. I should have known then that everyone has their own problems. I should have trusted in my friends not to judge me. But I couldn't think like that.

I tried to get on with work, but the customers were hard work now – I didn't have the patience to deal with them. When I almost felt like hitting some of them, I knew I was in trouble. When they had been frustrating or even mean before, I'd been able to deal with it. There had been so many times when someone had said something to me that I didn't like or agree with, but I had turned it around and still managed to sell them something! But now, I felt like I didn't even want to talk to them. And that wasn't a great way to make a living from engaging with people. I just couldn't help feeling like I had to get away from them.

In desperation, we decided to sell one of our two cars because money was so tight. But that was just a short-term fix. I knew that I had to find something else with a regular wage to take the pressure off the family, and especially off Michelle. So I ended up doing three jobs to make the same amount of money. It was really stressful. When I left my sales job, I felt bad for my boss who had treated me so well, but he knew some of what I was going through. He made it easy for me.

We drew on our family's support for childcare, and did what we could to keep our family afloat. After a few more months, Michelle got a lot more comfortable being back at work. Being around people she knew was good for her, even though no one on the team knew what she was going through. She worked in a large company where she dealt with customer complaints and trained colleagues. It was a stressful job, and loaded with pressures, but I think she liked that it got so busy – it meant that she didn't have to think about other things.

I found a new full-time sales job. I didn't have the same sense of purpose I'd had in my work before, but I started to earn a little more. Michelle's salary also increased, which meant that we were now back to a point where we had been before. It helped me feel better about coming home after work. Instead of feeling useless and worthless, I started to feel like I was pulling my weight again.

We were even able to go out as a couple sometimes. We took walks by ourselves, and really started talking again. It felt like it helped us work some things out. Being out in the open was like a special kind of therapy for us both. Sometimes we would take Ethan out with us, and start to feel like a normal family at last. At least, for those few precious moments.

Ethan was such an easy child to look after. Apart from that one night, he was as good as gold. He ate and slept on schedule, and he was always smiling. We were seeing him develop into a person before our eyes; his personality was starting to emerge, and he was such a joy to be with. He was learning how to walk, and starting to say a few things as well. Hearing him forming his first few words gave me goosebumps all over. It was so amazing watching him grow. I loved being a father, and when things were tough at work or at home, I would always try to think of him. He was my little saviour.

Ethan is completely unaware of the difficult times we experienced following his birth. He's full of life and energy, doing really well in school, and is very loving and sociable. The mother– father–son bond is strong and true, and I know it will stay like that forever.

No doubt, he'll become aware of the situation when he's older. We'll tell him when we feel he's ready to hear the truth. We understand that we need to be open about mental health with him, so that if he ever feels the way we felt, he knows that he can come to us and talk about it. I want him to understand that he is loved and accepted no matter what he goes through. He will grow up knowing that me and Michelle are always going to be here for him. I never want him to go through the kind of depression and loneliness I went through.

CHAPTER 11

In November 2005, we moved to a larger house, closer to my parents in Ogmore Valley, and, inevitably, it was pretty stressful. It made me never, ever want to move house again. We had to move out of our old house before the new house was ready, so we stayed with my parents for a bit – and we crammed in all our stuff too. The day we moved in was the day that George Best died – football always get in there somehow! By this time, we had a mountain of debt to repay, but the new house cost less so that helped us steady the ship a bit.

Michelle's mood was stable as Christmas approached. Along with the medication, she had been having some Cognitive Behavioural Therapy (CBT) group sessions. They really seemed to help her to stop her negative thoughts. Later, she taught me how to use the techniques too, and they really helped. I hadn't really talked to Michelle about how I had been feeling. But perhaps I didn't have to. She was my soulmate. If I was suffering, she instinctively seemed to know. So, without making a big deal out of it, she showed me how to rethink some of my negative thoughts.

Christmas in 2005 was so much better than the last one. We had a big new tree, and we decorated the house from top to bottom. I was looking forward to the family getting together and to having our first proper Christmas with Ethan. That last

Christmas definitely didn't count! I knew that Michelle wasn't completely recovered, and neither was I, but it was easy to forget all of that for a little while.

That Christmas was really all about taking stock of everything we had gone through, and reflecting on the important things. I was still worried about my own mood, but for those few days, I was just so grateful that Michelle had come out of the darkness into the light.

That Christmas spirit stayed with us long into the new year. So much had changed, but so much was just the same. I felt as if I had another chance to live the family life I'd been dreaming of. To come so close to losing the love of your life – and it really did feel like I was losing her – and then to get her back was the most amazing gift.

The drama around Ethan's birth had changed us. How could it not? But the positive events around Michelle's recovery changed us too. I had been feeling it for a while. I was starting to feel a lot less driven by money. I started to think seriously about jacking in my sales job, and doing something I really loved with my life. I had a family, a home, and I wanted this chance to do something meaningful. It was time to change tack. I wasn't interested in going through the motions of working from pay cheque to pay cheque, I wanted to try to do something meaningful with my life.

Over that year, I started getting involved in some voluntary work. Moving back to the valley where I was born turned out to be such a good move in so many ways. It meant I could engage in my own local community, and I started helping in the Wyndham Boys and Girls Club with the man / the legend ... Stan!

I had never forgotten how much Stan had helped me as a youngster, and I wanted to reciprocate his kindness. I had always loved being around Stan, who was always so positive. He was still just as much a role model to me now that he was in his seventies. The club needed a facelift for sure, but it was still the heart of the community. I knew all too well just how important it was for young people who didn't get on at school, and needed something else in their lives.

I loved that feeling of helping out and being a part of something bigger. And I yearned to do more. I thought about the support group Michelle had gone to, how it had helped her. I wanted to do the same for other people. So, in 2007, I started a community project in Bridgend. This was around the time when the media started reporting on the high number of suicides in the town. It was often sensationalist reporting, and did more harm than good for the families and communities around the borough of Bridgend. So our little charity gave the young people of Bridgend a safe space and, if they needed it, a friendly face to talk to.

I didn't know if it would do any good, and I didn't know if I would have the skills to make it work, but I really took to it. It felt like the missing piece of the jigsaw, so I started doing more, and looking for qualifications I could do to help me help others. The irony wasn't lost on me. After years of zoning out at school, and trying to get out of antenatal classes, I was finally volunteering to go back to school.

My confidence was growing, and it helped to silence some of those negative voices that had been telling me I was such a failure as a husband and father. Most of all, I enjoyed knowing I was making a difference to other people's lives. And the work we were doing was getting some great feedback. When I met with the kids in Bridgend, I couldn't help but be reminded of myself at that age. And after all the times when I felt like I'd let my younger self down, I knew I'd finally done something he'd have been proud of. I was giving the sort of help the younger me could have done with growing up.

The Williams family was going from strength to strength. Things weren't perfect, but they were normal. And normal felt great. Little Ethan was growing fast. You could see the confidence surging through him as he tried new things and really got to grips with his world. Above all, he had the one thing that we had always wanted for him – he was secure in the love of his parents.

I was really enjoying every aspect of fatherhood, and would take Ethan everywhere with me. I loved being around him and missed him so much when I was at work. Spending time with him helped take my mind off things.

Michelle didn't get better just like that. She never stopped working at getting better. Somehow, she juggled all the responsibilities of being a working mother and wife with always learning. Learning from everything she had experienced.

I was learning too. Michelle's illness and my involvement in the youth sector were developing my own interest in mental health issues. I started reading books about stress and anxiety and putting what I learnt into practice in my work in Bridgend. All that reading was good for me too. I was still having my bad days. There were times when all the old doubts came back, but, following Michelle's example, I kept working at it. I knew that self-managing my own mood was the best way for me to stay on top of it. Only now, "self-managing my anxiety" didn't come with a hangover the next morning!

If that makes it sound easy, it wasn't. And truth to tell, I was still keeping plenty of secrets. Looking back, I can't believe I was still hiding the truth about myself while helping others. It was daft that while I was trying to encourage kids in Bridgend to trust their mates, and to be open about what they were feeling, I was more tight-lipped than any of them. I was still locked in that old way of thinking that nobody would employ me if they knew what I was really thinking inside.

The years were starting to roll by in an easier fashion now. Deep inside, I knew that I still had some battles of my own to fight. But for now, at least, we were happy.

My mood was still up and down. I was doing things I loved with my life. And spending time with the people I loved. But after everything we had gone through, I was always on the lookout for signs of the old stress coming back. When it did, I sometimes faltered, and there were times when I'd give in and drink too much on the weekends, or sometimes even during the week.

In 2008, we finally managed to repay the mountain of debt we'd accumulated while we'd been dealing with Michelle's (and my own) illness. By now, we were starting to think of ourselves as survivors of this illness, not victims. Our marriage felt stronger than ever. We had coped with so much, and come through the other side. I didn't think anything could break us now.

CHAPTER 12

It doesn't matter how happy you are, or how contented; at some point, you always have to think about money. And by 2010, I was thinking about it a lot. Did we have enough to get by? I enjoyed focusing on the community work that I was doing, but I knew that my sales work was only just enough. And if I changed direction, like I wanted, it meant that I might earn even less. And I worried that it would take its toll on our family.

Michelle was already earning more than me, and I felt bad about that. Maybe it was old fashioned of me, but it was hard knowing that I wasn't the family's main breadwinner. As usual, Michelle tried to make it alright. She joked about it, and I'd laugh back, but it did affect me. I still wanted to be able to provide for my family, like I thought men were supposed to, and not being able to do that made me feel useless.

I was getting used to these feelings by now. It was a hard way to live life, always feeling like I was failing at being the best husband and father. And, in the end, that was my downfall.

This is a chapter in my life that I'm happy to talk about now, but for a long while, I really wasn't. I couldn't always face up to what I was going through, let along talk to anyone else about it. Eventually I learnt to embrace the fact that everyone gets ill. And I don't think there's a single person out there who is perfectly sane all the time. We all have issues, whether we bury them deep down, or allow ourselves to open up about them.

Without really acknowledging it, I had been ill for a while. And I had been getting more and more unhappy in the sales job I was doing at the time. But I needed my job to make me feel as though I was doing something worthwhile. I didn't feel like I could leave because I didn't think I'd find anywhere else that would pay me as well. I was really conflicted. I didn't know what to do.

There were times when I just couldn't face going in at all. I'd get up, get dressed, and leave in the morning to go to work ... and as far as Michelle was concerned, that's what happened. I'd come home and lie to Michelle that I had been working hard all day, when, really, I had simply sat inside my car and waited until it was time to go home. I was that desperate.

I hated that feeling of crippling insecurity. I couldn't bring myself to go to work and make the money we needed. I couldn't even tell Michelle what I was going through. It's only very recently that I've been able to open up to her about what I was doing. It turns out she knew all along.

Some days, I would just drive in any direction until I got tired. Sometimes I'd find somewhere quiet to eat, so I could just think. On the worst days, I would shop. The temporary high of spending money gave me a little lift. But like any high, it faded quickly, and when I came down from it, I'd feel miserable again. Worse, if I'd spent too much money. Work had always been something that I had identified myself with, but I had nothing left to identify with now. I wasn't very good at my job any more. I didn't believe in what I was doing. And I wasn't making any decent money.

I felt even worse knowing that Michelle was working so hard in her own job and I wasn't giving 100% in my own.

I'd known that this had been coming for a while. I'd been barely coping with all the feelings I'd been having since Ethan's birth. At best, I'd been keeping a lid on them. Trying everything I could to support Michelle.

I had tried to drown them in alcohol, trick them with my work in the community, and soothe them with love from my family. But I'd always known they'd catch up with me eventually.

Since it happened, I've found it easier to talk about depression honestly. But when people ask me what depression is, I still find it hard to explain. I suppose everyone has their own definition of it. Perhaps it's only something you can truly understand when you've gone through it. For me, it felt like I was on a treadmill, all day and all night, month after month, and no matter what I did, I couldn't get off. Everything was tiring. Everything felt like too much work. Nothing felt like it was enough. My life never felt like it was enough.

I never intended to take my life ... but could I have got to a point where I thought that was my only solution?

No. I couldn't have done that to Michelle and Ethan, not after everything we went through.

My grandfather on my mother's side passed away during the Christmas holiday. After seeing him alone on Christmas Day, I knew it was only a matter of hours before he departed. I could see it in his eyes; he was ready to leave us. I remember crying all the way home, and when I got there, I didn't tell Michelle what I had seen, or how it had made me feel. I didn't want to ruin her time.

The very next evening, he passed away. I couldn't get my head together until after the funeral. I remember wondering how Ethan was going to handle the death of a loved one at such a young age, but it turned out I should have been more worried about myself. Ethan, like always, took it in his stride.

So many people came to the funeral to pay their respects; my grandfather was loved by a lot of people. But it just brought home to me how real it all was. My grandfather's death had a huge impact on my mental health, but it was when Mam told me she had cancer that everything started to crumble at my feet. Hearing those words felt like a bomb going off in my head. I started to think the worst. That the woman who had brought me into this world was going to die. I felt cold all over, and numb to everything.

She told me the news so casually. She just dropped it into the conversation, like she was telling me about catching a cold. Mam told me that she was fine, and she never once felt sorry for herself. I think Dad moaned more about the weather than she did during her cancer treatment. I guess she just wanted to protect us from what she was going through.

It hit me really hard though. I had seen so many bad things happen in the hospital and I didn't want to go through anything like that with Mam. I wasn't just thinking of myself. It was going to affect everyone on such a huge scale. I thought of Mam as the woman who held the family together.

Those first few weeks were the hardest. Just like me, Mam didn't really open up about it. And for the first time, I knew how that made other people feel. It left me thinking the worst about what might happen. And because I was already feeling so bad, I inevitably thought the worst. My mind kept coming up with the cruellest, meanest things it could. And then I'd turn those fears over and over in my head.

Mum needed an operation. And it was almost impossible to cope with my worries in the days leading up to it. I prayed that everything would go to plan. I had started doing a lot of that.

The waiting was so stressful and I remember pacing around, not doing any work, not doing anything else. Just waiting and waiting and waiting for the call to come in.

I just couldn't face losing Mam. Not now. Not ever. I didn't have the skills to cope with the hole it would leave in our lives. But after two long years, more operations, and reconstructive surgery, she finally got the all clear.

No one could quite get over how she'd managed to stay so calm and relaxed during her treatment. I couldn't help but think about how brave she was, how strong she was. Even the staff at the hospital mentioned it. Mam is still such an inspirational figure to us all. She has helped so many people with her positive attitude to life, and she taught me such a valuable lesson. I learnt that whatever comes your way in life, you have to fight.

Everything that happened with Mam impacted on my work, and naturally, that impacted my income. I was still buying things secretly too, still trying to make myself happy by searching for value in material things.

Worse, I was starting to drink again. When the feelings got too much, and nothing else worked, it was all I could do to numb my feelings.

It was January. It was cold and it was dark, and I was struggling through the winter blues. Michelle and Ethan were always there – my beacons of hope. But work was almost impossible now. I found myself starting to cry without even feeling it creeping up on me. It was the worst I could ever remember feeling.

Ironically, while my mental health had deteriorated, physically I was in the best shape I'd been in for years. I was being careful about what I ate, and I was training hard every day for my black belt, and won the Welsh Championship in kickboxing for the over-35 age group.

But my mental health was sliding. And no sooner had I won than I just felt that overriding emptiness kick in all over again. It was just like all those shopping highs. As soon as they faded, I was left feeling lower than before. And the benefit of all those months of working hard, eating well, and training just drained away.

I just wanted to do nothing, and that made me feel guilty. I started to avoid people, stopped going to training sessions as much as I should, and started to eat rubbish food. I was coming apart.

I felt like I couldn't even express myself or make simple decisions. Just carrying on normal conversation was a struggle, never mind trying to close a sale. I wasn't just in a rut, I was about to lose my job, my company car, my wage.

I was ready to pack a bag and get out of Ogmore. It made perfect sense that I should go. I had become a liability. I didn't want to be around anyone, and I certainly didn't want Michelle and Ethan to see me like this. One dark day, at around 5pm, I phoned Michelle and I told her I couldn't do this any more. I headed straight to Coity Clinic, the adult mental health unit. All I wanted was to be admitted, but as I approached the door, I saw someone I knew and panicked. I couldn't let anyone know, so I turned and ran. I made it out of the hospital and sat under a tree sobbing. I just wanted the voices in my head to stop. I didn't know how to make them leave me alone. I wanted answers, but I didn't think I'd ever find them. I looked at my phone and saw that Michelle had phoned me five times. I wanted to phone her back, but I couldn't bring myself to do it. I felt like too big a failure.

Without thinking about what I was doing, I headed to an Irish bar in Bridgend, and just sat in the corner. And I stayed sitting there for five hours. I genuinely wondered if I should end my relationship with Michelle. I didn't want to. But I felt as if Ethan would be better off with someone else. Someone who could care for him and provide for him.

I didn't want to go home. I didn't want to go back there and let them all down again.

While I was in the pub, I started talking to a guy. I can't remember much of what we said, but I do know that he convinced me to go back home.

I don't know what happened next. I can't remember the next few days. But I knew I couldn't hide any more.

CHAPTER 13

I didn't know how to pick up the pieces of my life. So I focused on my family. It was the one thing I was sure of.

My relationship with Michelle and Ethan sustained me, but I was still uneasy about the future. I could feel sadness, frustration and anger rising in me, far too often. The bad days kept coming, and there didn't seem to be any good days any more. To get by in life, I did what everyone does in that situation – I hid my true feelings, and put on a smile.

I still wanted to find a different job. But it wasn't like the old days. I couldn't just walk out of one job and straight into another. Michelle continued to support me without ever making me feel inadequate. But I was getting so used to lying about my feelings that I started to lie to her too. I had never, ever wanted to do that to her knowingly. And I didn't mean to. But I wanted her to believe that everything was fine, when I knew that it wasn't. I still wanted to feel like I was protecting her. How I could I tell her that no matter how understanding she was, I still didn't feel better inside? That I was still just as scared underneath it all?

But no matter how good I thought I was being at keeping everything hidden, Michelle was better at reading my true feelings. She knew me far too well. She never confronted me, she didn't put any pressure on me, but it was clear that she knew I was hiding something from her. She simply waited for me to tell her when I was ready. And I think she sensed that day was coming.

I would have done almost anything to get rid of those feelings. It was like having a constant toothache. It made everything so unbearable. Some mornings, I couldn't be bothered to shower and then I felt disgusting. I stopped kickboxing, and I gave up on going for my black belt. I wasn't eating properly because my anxiety had given me stomach pains. So I was living off sugary drinks and coffee, and finding ways of having a drink in the house without getting caught.

Michelle would often ask me why other people never saw this side of me, and I never knew what to say to her. Was I so good at putting on the mask of happy-go-lucky Mark?

Weeks turned into months, and coping became my way of life. Because I couldn't imagine ever feeling normal again, I couldn't see any way out. As winter set in, things got even worse. I was going for walks on my own and having recurring thoughts of death and suicide. The idea of not having to live felt like a relief to me. It felt like my only way out. I wouldn't have cared if a bus hit me. I just didn't feel safe at all and didn't know how to deal with those feelings. I was thinking all sorts of things, and wondering how I would do it. And it just took me right back to the feelings I'd had after Ethan was born, and I was looking after Michelle.

I knew I needed to see a doctor; I felt like I was suffocating all the time. I couldn't even sit and watch TV. I didn't reply to emails or text messages or phone calls. I stopped everything. I became a complete stranger to myself. I wasn't the person I'd been before. And I wasn't yet the man I would become.

On the way to work with Michelle one day, the mask slipped, and I struggled to hold the emotion in check. I was trying desperately not to cry. As I dropped her off, she could see that something was very wrong. She didn't want to leave me. But I told her I was fine, I let her go, and then drove away.

I was sweating as I reached work. The pressure was building in my head. I could see my colleague; he was already getting customers over and selling like a pro. I felt numb. And I knew that day was going to be my last day in sales. I couldn't bear it any more. I never wanted to do it ever again.

I parked as far away from the front of the store as possible so that my colleague couldn't see me. I turned the car off, the engine fell silent. I felt a deep emptiness in me, my shoulders tensed, and my body felt tight. I couldn't get out of the car, let alone face trying to sell things to people and face getting rejected.

I started to cry, and I couldn't stop. I knew I couldn't leave the car in this state, so I took my phone and Googled 'mental health'. I found a number to call and hit it without thinking. I didn't know what I was going to say when the phone was picked up, but I needed to talk to someone. A lady answered after a few rings and didn't pressure me at all as she asked some questions. After speaking to her for a while, she told me to go straight to my GP. As I drove, I felt better as I turned away from the store, from my job.

Teary-eyed and confused, I told the doctor as much as I could. It was so odd finally telling someone other than Michelle about our journey here. I told him what had happened with Ethan's birth, and how that had made me feel. It had been five years at that point, but it still felt so fresh in my mind, with the added stress of losing so many people, of my job, of not feeling like myself. The doctor told me I was depressed. He prescribed some mild antidepressants and wrote me a sick note, which meant I no longer had to work.

I went onto Sickness Benefit; my £60 a week from the government was a huge comedown from my days as a sales manager, but I knew, deep down, that this was the way forward.

I told Michelle that I wasn't going back to that job, and I felt so much better after saying it. Maybe now I was finally going to get it all under control. But it meant that, at 37 years old, I was going to have to start my career all over again.

CHAPTER 14

Recovery takes time.

Those first few days after coming back from the doctors were the worst. I wanted to just lie down on my bed and not face the world, or anyone in it. I didn't know what my next move was going to be, or how I was going to get myself sorted. I remember that first day being horrific. After a few hours of just lying there, not moving, Ethan came home after school and I just held him, trying to take some value from everything we had gone through for him.

The more I wanted to be better, the more anxious I was about being better. My mind was playing tricks on me; whenever I felt like I was getting better, I would get a sense that it would never happen. The voices in my head would make me doubt myself. Sometimes, I would feel like giving into them. I was weak, and I would never recover from this.

I started driving out to the Bwlch Mountain, which was just a five-minute drive from my home. I would stand and look out towards the sea by Porthcawl. No matter what the day was like, I always looked at that view in shades of grey. Alone, by the edge of the mountain, I would wonder whether these feelings would ever stop.

I couldn't imagine how anyone would ever be able to cope with my mood swings. And the impulsive thoughts never stopped. I was scared for myself, and for everyone around me. I hadn't made plans to kill myself, but I couldn't say it would never happen. It felt wrong that I could think so dispassionately about ending my life. But I didn't recognise myself any more.

If I could have drunk myself into a coma, I would have done. I wanted to erase it all. But I never, ever stopped thinking about my family. I never, ever stopped believing in them. And that made it worse. Knowing all of that, and knowing how much they believed in me, made me hate myself even more.

I couldn't hide from reality forever. I got a call from a woman asking if I was coming back to work the next week. I said I wasn't sure, and she just asked me again, as though I'd given the wrong answer. So then I told her I wasn't coming back at all. I just couldn't face it. I had fought against it for too many years. It was time to stop.

Making that decision helped me to put other things into perspective. It was as if admitting to myself what the problem was helped me to take a bit more control of it. And that's when all the little changes started to build into something more significant.

Without the pressure to get up and go to work, I felt more able to look after myself a little bit better. Because I knew that getting up to shower wasn't the first stage of getting ready to go to work, I could do it. It was an ordeal though. We're just talking about getting up, getting into the shower and washing, but the effort made it feel like running a marathon with 100lbs on my back.

Slowly, I started to eat better. My runaway thoughts felt like they were slowing down, and I started to feel more like myself. I was still nowhere near the man I had been years before, but I was feeling far more positive about things in my life. The feeling of doom and despair that had hovered over my head for the best part of five years was slowly fading.

I started to find more value in taking time out and relaxing. Instead of fixating on the bad things I had no control over, by obsessing over all the bad things that were happening in the world, I did things that would make me feel better.

As the days turned into weeks, I opened up to Michelle about everything. I told her how I'd been feeling. I told her I was sorry, that I'd try harder to be a better husband. I let it all pour out. All the pain, all the fear and all the regret ...

Michelle didn't judge me for any of it. She just listened. And that was all I needed.

After I'd stopped working out in the gym, I'd stopped exercising altogether. So, with Michelle's help, I learnt some very simple exercises that helped to improve my mood. I learnt the art of mindfulness. I'd start by sitting comfortably somewhere and breathing slowly, listening to the sounds I was making. I would then visualise blowing a candle very gently – just enough to make the flame flicker, and then focus in on the change in my breathing. I was giving my mind a rest as well as my body, and I was starting to feel the benefits of becoming more aware of the things they were trying to tell me.

I found a counselling service called Guiding Stars, and met a woman called Sarah who helped me to get a more objective sense of my life. I started on an eight-week mindfulness course with an amazing teacher in Bridgend. I was starting to really see the effects of thinking in different ways. It wasn't all about positive thinking, it was more about considering problems and life situations in different ways than I was used to. It helped me to focus better on things, so that my mind didn't feel so floaty as it had before. I was learning skills that helped me cope with everyday life. I was better with Ethan too. For once, I really felt as if I was giving him my full attention.

I felt that my depression was lifting. I was embracing my new passion for life. I changed my thoughts, I changed my mind, and I was looking forward to the future, which only weeks ago seemed so far away.

As time passed, I started to wake up better in the morning. I started to appreciate all the good things in my life. I even started to sing in the shower. That might not have been music to Michelle's ears, but to me it said something really significant about how much I'd improved. I started to look at the problems in my life in a more objective way, so that instead of focusing on the worst-case scenarios, I started thinking in terms of alternative solutions. I noticed that my posture changed too. As all the pent-up pain and anxiety started to leave my body, I found myself standing straighter and walking taller. I stopped shouting, because, ever-so-slowly, I had less to be angry about. I didn't feel the same relentless need to criticise other people.

I was becoming more aware of my own failings though ...

I had passed a life coaching course before I had collapsed under the weight of my depression, and I know that helped me a lot in knowing how to restructure my life. But I also knew that something was still holding me back: my drinking. And it was dawning on me that unless I could tackle that, I wasn't ever going to get any better.

It was my coping mechanism, pure and simple. But it was dangerous, and it was destructive. I talked to Michelle about it openly, and she was keen that I should see a professional about it.

I was so nervous for my first appointment. Even though I knew I needed it, part of me still wondered if I was really that bad. Everyone had their coping mechanisms, didn't they? The more I questioned myself, the more I nearly talked myself out of it. And I know I'd repeated that pattern before – when I'd talked Michelle out of staying in hospital, and when I'd backed out of admitting myself for treatment. I tried rationalising it by thinking that I might be taking the place of someone who needed it way more than I did. But I held my nerve and sat down with the counsellor, Dave, who was very down-to-earth. He explained everything before we got started, and reassured me that everything we spoke about would be kept between us. I didn't feel judged, so I felt I was able to talk openly.

I told him about how I thought I had got myself into this state. Over the next few sessions, Dave taught me some coping skills, helping me to challenge negative thoughts whenever they intruded. I came away feeling like a brand-new person. I couldn't get away from the fact that I still had issues in my life that made me drink and shop. I knew that I had come to place too much importance on material things, and I understood the patterns of behaviour that made me buy things for myself when times were hard. But with Dave's help – and Michelle's – I felt like I now had the tools to deal with those feelings.

As the days passed, I was learning more and more about mental health issues – not just my own. I was reading and listening to as many different people as I could, learning about the reasons why people became depressed, from outside influences, to personal insecurities, to chemical imbalances in their brains.

I was also learning about Cognitive Behavioural Therapy (CBT) which Michelle had told me about when she had been getting support for her PND, and I was applying it to my own life, to help me deal with the negative feelings I'd had for years. I started to learn how different environments and different situations impacted me, and how I could cope with them. I also found that music was a great help. It helped me focus, and banish some or all of the negative thoughts.

Over the last few months, I had been noticing that I'd been getting mysterious body pains. It wasn't related to exercise. I later found out that physical symptoms are commonly seen in individuals with depression. Aches and pains are sometimes the first symptoms, and can include chronic pain in the limbs, joints, and back. A significant number of people with depression who seek treatment only tell their doctors about the physical symptoms, not the mental or emotional ones. This can make a diagnosis very difficult.

I was on my way to another diagnosis though. I was being cared for under the Community Mental Health Teams at the time, which would later lead me to the diagnosis of Attention Deficit Hyperactivity Disorder (ADHD) which I had been self-managing all these years.

As I come out of my own depression, I realised more and more just how much Michelle had done for me. She had been through so much herself, and yet she had always stood by me. She understood me so well and seemed, instinctively, to know what I was feeling. All of these realisations – and all of this gratitude – helped me to see everything more clearly, and the one thing that I saw, above all else, was just how much Michelle meant to me.

I still felt as if I was in recovery – and I was still on antidepressants – but I was starting to find the idea of work more appealing again. But I knew that I could never put myself in a pressurised, target-based workplace environment ever again. I got an interview for a job in a hospital, working with patients with personality disorders on a forensic ward. It was the first time that I'd be going to work on medication. I didn't know how I was going to be able to handle that, or how my managers were going to see that. I thought it was best to be totally up-front with them, so I told them about my situation from the start. Fortunately, they understood. They told me it didn't matter, and reassured me that, of all people, those working in mental health would understand.

Everything starts with change.

I used to be terrified of change. I worried that I could never be the same person if I embraced it. As if my identity was so fragile that it would get lost in the transition. But I was starting to realise that if you're brave enough, there can be so many better opportunities out there to investigate.

It was time to embrace the fear and embrace the possibility of change.

I got the job.

That was obviously a huge change and a massive step forward in my recovery. But looking back, I knew that it had been all the little changes that had helped lead me there. Like drops of water turning into a flood, the little steps had all helped build my sense of achievement and confidence, which had made me ready to apply for that job.

I carried on working with Sarah. She quickly realised that I'm a visual and kinaesthetic learner, and saw that, for me, tapping into different ways of learning and therapy helped me to open up more about my feelings.

After six months of engaging on my own path to recovery, and of Michelle looking after me, her own depression came back.

I can't describe how I felt when I saw that happen, when the depression crept back into her. I hated feeling as if we had gone through everything that we'd gone through, only for it to come back so easily. It was as if it had never gone away at all.

Suddenly, the roles were reversed. When Michelle started to feel unwell, I resumed the role of caring for her. That familiar, haunted look was back in her eyes.

Times had changed, so we didn't just rely on the support from the NHS. We looked to the internet for new ideas, and picked up books on dealing with depression. I was clinging on to any hope, any possibility. We even started to do yoga in the front room. Our neighbours were probably wondering what on earth we were doing!

I would have sold everything we had to make sure she was well again.

After everything we had learnt, we were able to manage the depression a bit more easily this time. Michelle called in sick, and we made sure she took enough time off to make herself better. That was hard though. Her employer wanted her to return as soon as possible because she was so missed. She took up the offer of occupational therapy that her employer arranged, which included four counselling sessions. She engaged really well, and it definitely helped, but when it ran out, we had to find another counsellor; we didn't want to end up going backwards.

Michelle spent a few weeks with her mum. I wanted her with me, but I knew that the peace and quiet would do her good. My parents helped me care for Ethan, and between us all, we got through it. We had learnt from our experiences and we moved on all the stronger.

CHAPTER 15

Things weren't perfect, but they didn't need to be. We felt more secure than we had for a long time.

I had started going back to the gym regularly again, and while I was working out one day, I started talking to a guy called Brian. My first thought when I saw him – which was probably the same thought a lot of people had – was that I would never want to pick a fight with him! But something inside me made me talk to him. After we'd been talking a little while, he mentioned that he had to go to the PRAM (Perinatal Response and Management Service) group in Bridgend with his wife. A group for women with PND. He told me that his wife had postnatal depression and that the group was helping her to get through it.

I listened intently to what he said about the group. He told me that it was run entirely by the NHS, and that a lady named Gail ran it and helped everyone there. Later, I would find out that Gail was the same community practice nurse who had helped me and Michelle so much.

Within a few minutes of him telling me that, I had told him everything about me. It was a strange scene – us two manly guys, standing by the weights, talking about our feelings! Not something I'd have been able to do a year or two earlier. I couldn't believe that I had told this complete and utter stranger more than I had said to my best friends. But I knew that he would really understand and, for some reason, I put all my trust and faith in him.

Brian had been in the building trade for the last 32 years of his life. He was a proper man's man, and yet he was completely fine with opening up to me about his feelings. He had battled many things in his life, and when his wonderful wife had PND, he'd nursed her, and managed to look after his daughter at the same time. Once his wife became more able to cope, he had experienced a complete breakdown. His world became a dark place, and he didn't know how to cope with anything. It was like hearing my own story told back at me.

We started to talk more about what we had both felt, about what we had gone through, and about all the ways it had affected us. Neither of us had had a diagnosis of PND – I don't think too many dads would have had that diagnosis back then. But a look passed between us that said it all. *We* knew. And we both agreed that there needed to be more support out there for men who had experienced PND. It seemed so wrong. Nothing had changed in the last few years. We had made huge advances in technology, and yet we had slipped on so many of the important things in life. I had now met a couple of guys within the space of just a couple of miles of home who had both experienced PND. And they were the ones who were willing to talk about it. On that evidence, I knew there must be thousands more.

When I went home that evening, I started to look for websites with information on men's groups for PND, but I couldn't find anything. There was nothing on how to support a partner with PND, or anything about what to do if you experienced PND as a man. I was completely shocked. I knew how much value that would have had for me. Perhaps if I'd had that level of support, I wouldn't have suffered for six years. And I wouldn't have felt like I was all alone.

My entire life changed from that realisation. With so much going around my head, I couldn't get to sleep that night. There was too much to think about. How many more fathers were suffering out there? I felt at once excited and angry and nervous, all at the same time. I knew there was an opportunity to do something really significant here. The next day, I went back to the mental health centre where they had helped me a few weeks before. I was nervous about it at first – there was a very real possibility that they would just laugh at me. But after thirty minutes of thinking about it, I just walked towards it.

A woman invited me into the back office to discuss my concerns. As I briefly told her my idea, I could see by her reaction that I might be onto something. She asked me to come back and meet with her again, along with another lady. We booked the meeting for the next day, and I was so eager to impress I turned up early.

When I was introduced to the support worker, I realised that it was the same woman who had talked to me over the phone when I was in the car at my lowest ebb. I told them why I was so sure we needed to build a support group to help fathers like me and Brian.

I was so excited when I got home that night. Michelle and I started to think of a name for the group, and Michelle suggested the name "Fathers Reaching Out". As soon as the name left her lips, I knew that was the one.

I went into workaholic mode, maybe for the first time in my life. I was so interested in finding out everything I could about postnatal depression, but there was so little out there.

Initially, Fathers Reaching Out was intended to support fathers when their partners were going through postnatal depression, but it turned out to have a bigger remit than that. I was still learning too …

When I had been diagnosed with depression, my Doctor hadn't gone into detail. He certainly hadn't suggested that my experience might have been the result of post-traumatic stress disorder from seeing Michelle being cut open in the labour ward. But, after a couple of months running Fathers Reaching Out, I had probably picked up more understanding of male PND than most doctors would have had at that time.

So many things made sense to me now. I had always been so afraid of losing loved ones. That night in the maternity ward, I really thought I was going to lose Michelle. Maybe even Ethan. The shock of that night had lain dormant for weeks, months and years, and then, when the stress of our lives had caught up with me, all that stress took over.

I remember the first meeting I set up in Bridgend. I didn't know who was going to turn up or how it was going to go. I had no funding, but I was lucky to have the room for free. I had tried not to worry too much about it, or else I might not have been able to go through with it. I was acting on my promise to myself to embrace new possibilities.

As the night started, around six fathers turned up from all over, but mostly from where I lived. We sat around a table and I explained how the organisation had started, and what we had planned for the future. I was taken aback by how quickly the men opened up after I had told them about my own struggles.

It wasn't just me leading the group: a counsellor, Sue Moet, sat in with us and was pretty much amazing as she explained how she could help. I didn't know if I'd be seeing any of the guys again, so I made sure that they all had support when they left, including the free service that Sue was providing.

I didn't know if there would be a next time, so I was amazed when, after the two-hour session, everyone wanted to meet again the following week. I had planned for monthly meetings, but clearly the group was working. I was beyond happy. There was lots to do. I knew that I needed to expand my own knowledge, particularly about perinatal mental health, covering pre and postnatal depression, as well as anxiety.

It wasn't long before I was encouraged to tell my story to the local press. They said it would elevate my presence and help promote the work we were doing. We needed to get the word out there. So I did the interview. And just like that, things went crazy. The national press for Wales phoned up, and said they wanted to do a piece on me and Michelle, and our journey so far.

As a result of that, I was put in touch with Dr Jane Hanley, who would quickly become my new mentor and friend – an extraordinary woman who had written the essential book on perinatal mental health for professionals. She was so down-to-earth, and we quickly bonded because of our passion for creating awareness of perinatal mental health for fathers. She had recently produced a film with Boyd Clarke, the famous Welsh actor, about the importance of fatherhood, and she spoke so passionately about it.

Within weeks, she was training me up in perinatal mental health and gave me the confidence to talk about it with more authority. I learnt more about the differing experiences of fathers who suffered with PND, and about what happened after the fact as well.

I felt like I had a purpose now. I had found what I wanted to do with my life; this was what I was meant to be doing, and I know that it helped with my own recovery. Listening to other people's stories and helping them felt good; it felt right.

At first, I was more than happy for it to be a local thing, but as soon as it started to grow nationally, I knew that I wanted every single father in the country to have what we had; a simple but effective support network. And the requests for personal appearances and media shots were coming in ...

I was invited onto Radio 4's *Women's Hour* to discuss my story, and to discuss the issue of male PND. It was a big step up from talking to small groups of people about the subject, but it was a wonderful platform for me to really raise the stakes. Despite my nerves, I found that I enjoyed speaking out on the subject. My mission to embrace new opportunities had carried me this far, and I wasn't going to turn my back on any chance to raise more awareness.

With the groups now expanding all over Wales, and with free rooms given to us by organisations, I was getting calls to set up similar sessions in other parts of the country. By doing it voluntarily, I was now giving up my own income to make sure fathers were being supported. Sometimes, it would be over the phone, other times via social media and email. But it was getting too big and with very little help, I found it hard to operate on my own.

There was also the pressure of making a living and paying the mortgage. Just like before, our bills were becoming too much to handle. I knew that it was time to move into a different role – to become an even more active campaigner – so that I could help spearhead the changes we needed to make to get this movement growing …

I sought out new partner organisations that already had a support network around the country that I could simply tap into. I had a few meetings and, without too much difficulty, a national charity took us on. It seemed like there was a real appetite for more knowledge and understanding around the issue.

And the more we did, the more we found there was to do. I kept meeting more and more fathers whose own experiences helped shape what we did. I met a father who talked to me about his experience of PTSD after childbirth. It wasn't something that people were really speaking about enough outside of our circles. I started to meet mothers who said that their partners didn't want to talk about the childbirth, and fathers who said that it had traumatised them. But it was only really after speaking to this one father that I knew I had to do something.

I had spoken openly on my struggles about seeing Michelle go through the C-section, and about how we really hadn't known what to expect. Unsurprisingly, I wasn't alone. There were fathers who had gone through the same thing as me, or who had lost their babies. There were mothers who were suffering from the memories of C-sections that still haunted them. We had gone through so many of these things ourselves.

One father told me that he had witnessed his wife die and then come back, and then have the emergency team rush in. He was told to leave while they tried to resuscitate her, and was left on his own for an hour without any kind of explanation as to what was happening. His newborn son was born with a lack of oxygen and then had to be put on an emergency unit, but he only found out after the fact. He told me that extreme anxiety set in at this point and he felt faint. Everything turned out fine at the hospital, but it was when his partner confessed to wanting another child that it all turned bad. They started fighting, and it felt as if neither of them could understand the other any more. Sadly, in the end, they split up. His life disintegrated: he started drinking and then lost his job as a result. Afterwards, he suffered with nightmares and flashbacks, and he had begun to feel panicky around other people. He, like me, never told anyone.

I told him that he needed to talk to his partner about everything; that he needed to be honest and open with her. I told him how I had my own triggers, that certain smells and music could bring it all back for me. It was easy now to be absolutely open and honest about my experiences – and it made interacting with people so much easier. No one ever laughed at me. No one tried to marginalise my feelings. I just met men and women who were interested and supportive.

I don't know what happened to him after. I hope he managed to work things out with his wife.

So many of the men I met told me how their relationships, which were fine before the illness, had disintegrated after. They said that everything was "perfect" before, but then everything changed. I recognised so much of my life in their experiences

So many new fathers just didn't know how to look after their partners as well as their new baby, and still tried to do everything they were doing before. They described the anxiety they felt, the stress, and the pressure. Some of them spoke about the horrific scenes they saw in the operating theatre, and about the birth complications they had gone through. Everyone had their own story to tell.

Many of the fathers I spoke to were first-time fathers, and they felt like their identity had changed because of it. They no longer felt like the same person they had been before. They were something new, something different. They felt like they had to stay in jobs, which they felt trapped in, and they felt useless at home.

Everyone I spoke to agreed that they had struggled to tell anyone how they felt. They didn't know if anyone would ever understand. They worried that the social services might become involved if they weren't careful and if they didn't try to show that everything was fine. I had been so lucky to have had the support of my family. Some of the men I spoke to hadn't even had that. They had been completely alone. They gave up on work, bringing on financial difficulties. And just like me, they drank to try to cope with it all.

In our own lives, we were coping better than ever. By the end of 2012, it felt as if Michelle was completely recovered. She juggled her work role with motherhood beautifully. My own working life was more complicated. If I'd had the opportunity to devote all of my time and attention to the support group – and all the publicity – I could and would have done. But I still needed to provide for my family. I was working with people who had committed criminal offences, and who had personality disorders. It could be very, very difficult. The stress of being in such an environment reached a high one day when one of the patients started acting aggressively towards everyone. I was trying to calm him down, as I had a good relationship with him, but then he said, 'I'm going to rape your wife.'

I remember being very still for a second or two. And then I just exploded. I shouted at him, telling him that he would never even get close to my wife. I fought the urge to hit him; I had never felt so angry before. But I dug deep and walked away quite calmly. My life had improved in so many ways that I had the capacity to deal with stress in a new way.

CHAPTER 16

Fathers Reaching Out had reached out further than I'd ever imagined. I was getting calls and enquiries from all over the world. I was invited to appear on a BBC Wales programme with Michelle so that we could talk about our experiences of PND. We were getting quite used to telling our stories. How far we'd come from those two people who couldn't bring ourselves to say anything about our experiences.

While we were filming, I got two more calls; one was from Mind, the mental health charity, telling me that I had been shortlisted for the Mind Media Awards in London, which would be hosted by Stephen Fry. The second was to tell me I had been shortlisted for the Local Hero award at the Pride of Britain Awards. I couldn't quite believe it. It had only been eight months since our journey with Fathers Reaching Out had started.

I had watched the Pride of Britain Awards every year, never with a dry eye, and I couldn't quite believe that I was going to be a part of it, particularly when they invited me to do a little filming for them.

They put us up in a lovely hotel, and I remember sitting on the bed, not being able to believe where we were, or what was about to happen. I couldn't believe that I was about to be rubbing shoulders with television celebrities and so many other famous people.

We put on our best clothes, and headed to Grosvenor House in a limo laid on for us. We were so nervous as we were driven there; we had no idea what was going to happen. We walked on the red carpet, and the flashes from the paparazzi were everywhere. We just let them tell us where to stand and how to pose, and tried to take it all in as the white light of their cameras lit up the October night.

I could barely believe that I was surrounded by so many people who had done so many great things with their lives. I was on my very best behaviour, and although I drank a little wine, I kept myself in check. The last thing I wanted to do was make a fool of myself now that I was hobnobbing with TV stars. I remember sitting next to the football pundits and the England football manager at the time, Roy Hodgson. Even though of course I am Welsh, it still gave me goosebumps. To think that a boy from the Valleys, who was told once that he wouldn't do anything in life, was now being called a local hero at one of the biggest events in the United Kingdom.

And then they counted the votes, and revealed that I hadn't won! I was over the moon just to be crowned Welsh Local Hero, and experience something that money simply can't buy. I looked at Michelle and could see that something that had been so bad in our lives had turned into something good.

Afterwards, I spoke with people from all walks of life and knew that I was onto something that needed to change, not just in the United Kingdom, but all around the world. It felt so amazing to speak to people who had done amazing things and feel as if they appreciated my work too.

When I think back to it now, I still feel like pinching myself. But if I'm honest, the very the best part of the whole thing wasn't the glitz and the glamour, or the posh hotels and the celebs ... it was the renewed sense of purpose I felt when I got home. I felt inspired by the people I had seen, and was so motivated to keep doing more. One thing I will always remember was meeting

Stephen Hawking with Michelle – the photo of the three of us sits proudly on our wall.

After the Pride of Britain Awards, I was really trying to push out awareness in any way I could. I wish that I'd had the funding to make it easier, but as it was, I was completely out of pocket every single month. I even hid money from Michelle to make it happen, and that didn't sit right with me. After all, people were spending thousands in other sectors, I wanted us to compete as best we could.

Never a day went by when I wasn't reminded of just how important the work was. I was receiving countless emails from families and people that needed help. I knew that I needed to keep doing everything I could to get the message out there ...

I sent pitches to magazines and blogs, writing for as many people as I could. I took out adverts, and even paid for a big billboard promoting the importance of fathers' mental health in the middle of Cardiff. That was the biggest thing I ever did, and the reaction was exactly what I wanted. If things had been just busy before that, they snowballed afterwards. Emails and enquiries started flooding in from all over the world.

Suddenly it felt like everyone was talking about fathers and perinatal mental health. One of my proudest moments was becoming a plenary speaker for the International Marce Society, which produced research for perinatal mental health. I spoke in front of footballers and rugby league players, and explained why mental health was just as important as physical wellbeing. I hope that I got through to them.

In 2013, a new organisation called "How is Dad Going" launched in Australia. They wanted to start a similar thing to Fathers Reaching Out and asked me for my story. I was more than happy to help; I couldn't believe how fast things were moving around the world.

After networking and socialising with professionals in the sector, I started to realise how much I enjoyed doing this work. It all helped me to feel so much better about myself. But it could be draining at times. What little funding we had wasn't enough. And coming to terms with the fact that we could never do everything we wanted was always difficult. Over the next couple of years, I had to keep fighting for more money. There were times when it felt like I had secured more funding, and then offers dried up, or disappeared. Having coped with depression, it was tough taking on all that extra disappointment.

The requests for appearances continued, and I felt as if Fathers Reaching Out had really played the crucial part in developing greater understanding of fathers' pre and postnatal mental health all around the world. I was being asked for interviews from magazine companies from across the world, speaking to professors and doctors, and, best of all, receiving calls from people who thanked me for my help and my research.

I was even asked to do an educational video with Denise Welch from *Coronation Street*, *EastEnders*, and *Loose Women*. We met in Liverpool, and she told her story, not as a much-loved celebrity, but as a woman – as Denise. We were hanging on her every word, and, as she finished, there was a little moment's silence; we had been so touched by everything she'd said. Despite her infinitely busy schedule, she gave her time so generously.

The film we both appeared in highlighted our experiences of depression, but considered it from the professional's perspective too. The aim was not simply to get people to listen, but also to educate and teach them as much as we could.

My profile had been steadily building, but that film took it all to a whole other level. Suddenly, I was becoming more and more recognisable. I was a little bit worried about Michelle and Ethan, how the media would consume and portray them. I wanted to protect them from all of that, especially considering everything that had happened with Michelle. Her story of what she went through was her own to tell, on her own terms.

I was invited to appear on BBC *Breakfast* with Jeszemma Garratt from the Fatherhood Institute, an organisation that talks about the importance fatherhood and strives to increase services for parents. It helped promote the message that everyone needs supporting, and how fathers didn't need to suffer in silence. I was so happy to be taking part, because I knew that it was going to be broadcast nationally and would bring in even more awareness. The response was hugely welcoming, and I'm so glad I was able to do it.

Within days, I was in demand again. I was asked if I could be involved with the National Childbirth Trust for new research they had coming out in 2015. The people working on the research were more than eager to hear what I had to say about fathers with PND. And I saw that they had the same visions as me, of wanting to support as many people as possible.

The report showed that over a third of fathers were worried about their own mental health, and over 70% of them were worried about their partner's mental health. I couldn't believe how high the numbers really were. But when I thought back to the meetings I had taken part in, and all the fathers I had met and spoken to, I realised that it really was true.

I'm so proud of having been involved in that report. It's so important that the research is out there and freely available for people to read and to see for themselves that this problem is so much bigger than it had ever been portrayed before. In many ways this was like a culmination of all the work I'd been doing, and it felt like one of the proudest moments of my life. Straightaway, I knew just how much of an impact it was going to have.

The launch of the report was embargoed until Father's Day, and the week leading up to it went so slowly for me; I couldn't wait for people to hear about it. When the launch came, I was invited to go on *Good Morning Britain* with Michelle, as well as the BBC *Breakfast* show on Father's Day with Dr Anna Machin. They even put me and Ethan up in Manchester in a fancy hotel suite the night before the show.

The media got hold of the research and the story spread quickly. People around the UK started talking about the report, about the research, and about the charities involved in it.

By the end of that week, I was completely shattered, and I was glad when the final broadcast was done the following Sunday. The momentum had been building for so long, and now it felt like we had really achieved something truly significant.

CHAPTER 17

The more you achieve, the more you want to achieve. And I wasn't finished with my ambitions for Fathers Reaching Out yet. I remember seeing an advert for a silly awareness day in a newspaper and thinking how meaningless it was. Certainly nothing like as important as Fathers Reaching Out.

And that's when it occurred to me: I needed to make this into a national awareness day.

I had a quick Google to see if there was anything like that already out there, and I wasn't surprised to discover there was nothing. Straightaway, the ideas started to spark in my mind, and I knew that this was what I wanted to do ...

It made perfect sense to schedule it the day after Father's Day, the Monday after the Sunday. It took some doing, but we had a great team, and we all pulled together to start campaigning and raising awareness of what we wanted to do.

I got busy on social media, asking people who had helped me in the past to get the message out there, and we started blogging our ideas for the day. Because we'd managed to raise our profile so much, it wasn't too difficult to get the support of some of the mental health charities, and everyone we spoke to gave us all the help and encouragement they could.

The message kept coming back to me loud and clear: we need this day! We all need to acknowledge these issues. Stuff pancake day, give us a father's mental health day!

Although most of us – men and women alike – are socialised to think of men as providers of support during the perinatal period and early parenthood, a wealth of research shows that 10% of new dads experience paternal postpartum depression (up to 50% when mum is depressed)! And they need support of their own. One of the most important things I learnt was there isn't just one reason for depression in the postnatal period – there are often so many factors involved.

I knew we needed a day to make people understand just how bad the problem was, but also to give all parents and professionals access to more resources and useful information.

I wanted the day to follow straight on after Father's Day in the UK. I know that not all fathers are happy following what is supposed to be a happy Father's Day. And with suicide rates so high among men, I wanted fathers and organisations to blog about the day each year.

I thought the first day was going to start small – I thought that if we got a few people talking on social media we'd be doing fine. But I should have learnt not to think so small ...

The day completely exploded and organisations around the world wanted to support us. The second year was even better, with so many amazing, passionate people telling their stories and getting involved. I was having conversations with people all over the world telling me how desperately they needed support in their own countries. Professionals were weighing in with their research too. The incredible support we received proved just how badly we needed this awareness-raising day.

More radio appearances were followed by more podcasts, and everything we did just helped raise our profile. We still didn't have any money – just a logo – but there was such a huge appetite for this message that everything just took off.

The day wasn't just about raising awareness; we had some practical goals too. From the start we had been campaigning to change the NICE guidelines to reflect the reality of the male PND experience, and getting heaps of support behind our #HowAreYouDad campaign. My Member of Parliament for Ogmore, Chris Elmore, even called for a debate in Parliament. One of our biggest achievements was getting our story on the BBC News site about screening fathers as well as mothers. From my own experience, and the stories of countless others, I knew that far too many men are not diagnosed during the postnatal period. I was so pleased to see comments praising me for opening up about my journey and for being brave enough to say how I'd been feeling. At the time of writing, the story is still available to view, and continues to draw new supporters and give hope to dads who have been experiencing PND.

Our third year was bigger again. We got some more of the most respected thinkers on male PND behind us, with the likes of psychologists Dr Daniel Singley from California and Dr Andrew Mayers. The day keeps on growing and I am confident now that it will go on getting bigger and reaching further than ever before. And about time too: it's estimated that there are more than 13 million fathers suffering with PND worldwide each year.

As our international reach grew, I started to accept a few offers to make public appearances overseas. I was invited to speak at the International Marce Society (for perinatal mental health) in Melbourne, and was waiting at the airport when I received two very significant phone calls ...

The first was an invitation to the Mind Media Awards, after a documentary I was involved in was nominated. And the second was from Heads Together, the Royal Family charity!

I sat in the lounge at Heathrow and phoned Michelle, telling her what had happened, but that we couldn't tell anyone at all.

We were going to meet Prince William, Kate, and Harry! I could barely believe what was happening.

But first, I had to travel to Melbourne. When I arrived there, half a world away from everything I knew, I felt isolated and lonely. Of course, so much had been happening over the last few years; we had come so far in such a short space of time, it wouldn't have been surprising if I had been feeling burnt out. I checked into my hotel and stayed in the room, feeling lower than I'd felt for a very long time. I missed Michelle and Ethan very badly.

On the morning of the conference, I was interviewed for an Australian radio show. I was telling my story to a whole new audience, and in a country where, perhaps, the male identity is even more strongly defined than in the UK. They were interested in my story, and they really wanted to know about everything I had done in the name of mental health support for fathers.

After the interview, I headed to the conference. I was already feeling pretty stressed about the time I had been assigned to talk. They had only given me 10 minutes, but all my other talks had been between 30 and 40 minutes. I didn't know how I was going to be able to put everything into such a small amount of time.

I got up on the stage and made sure that I highlighted the most important parts within a few minutes. I quickly started to feel at ease and got into my flow. I couldn't believe that the little boy from Ogmore Valley, who had left school with nothing, was now speaking to an international audience, alongside all these professionals. I think I was the only person who had no letters after their name on that stage, but my own experience and the information I had gathered from fathers over the years proved to be more than enough.

When I left the stage, I was extremely proud. I felt vindicated. And I knew that my experience – and all of the other experiences that had been relayed to me – mattered. Through all the hurt and pain we had gone through, this was what truly mattered.

That night, I was desperate to reach out to Michelle and Ethan and tell them I'd done it, and to celebrate my achievement with them. They were so pleased for me and couldn't wait for me to get back home. I couldn't wait to go home either, and I knew that very soon, my little family would be going to meet the Royals!

When the big day came, we headed to London as early as we could. We wanted to make the most of the day and the experience. We headed towards County Hall, next to the London Eye. A lady talked us through details of the day and asked us if we wanted to do a film about our journey, and, of course, we said yes. What a way to keep our memories alive! And then she told us that we were going to have a 10-minute chat with the Prince himself. We could barely believe it.

The room soon started to fill with other people, who all had incredible stories to tell. There were people from all over the country, people who ran huge organisations, people who were doing so many great things, all in the name of mental health. I spoke to as many people as I could, telling them about the importance of fatherhood and mental health. And everyone I spoke to seemed to agree with what I had to say.

It's so surreal meeting someone from royalty, and coming face to face with people who you have only ever seen on the TV. The effect they have on a room when they walk in really is something to behold. Though I pride myself on being able to speak to anyone, that moment showed me that even I had my limits. I could barely muster up the bravery I needed to walk over to him. We literally didn't know how to walk up to him and speak to him. But then someone formally introduced us and suddenly, there we were: me, Michelle, and Prince William.

I could barely believe it and, even now looking back, I still get shivers thinking about it.

The main event was hearing Prince William give his speech about how he was going to change the stigma around mental health. Seeing all three of them up there – William, Kate, and

Harry – I was just covered in goosebumps. We were part of something special, Michelle and I. Together it felt like we were going to change lives forever. And soon after that, I received a phone call inviting me to speak on mental health for fathers in Parliament in December of that year.

Everything felt like it was really coming together now. It all just seemed so ... perfect. I don't think I'd ever thought life could get any better ...

As Christmas came and went, I was invited to get involved with *Out of the Blue* films by the Best Beginning charity. So I went to London to talk about my struggles, and it felt like I was being presented as the spokesperson for all the fathers who had been through this – and that's what made the work we did so powerful. We made some excellent films and apps, and I was really proud of the work. It just showed the power you can have when you're open and honest about things. I knew it would get people talking, and get more fathers to open up and get the help they needed. And just to add the finishing touch, the Duchess of Cambridge herself was going to make a presentation for *Out of the Blue*, and I was invited to go along and meet her.

The launch was absolutely incredible; I was so honoured to meet the Duchess of Cambridge. Her speech about how we needed to fight stigma for this generation, and the generations that were to come felt like it truly came from the heart.

I know that these are things that I'm going to tell the grandchildren about. Everything that had happened was going to become a story to tell for years to come. It gave me a different perspective on things – maybe, just maybe, the pain that me and Michelle had endured had been worthwhile if this was the life it had brought to me.

I was really feeling on top of the world now. On a personal level, it was good to think that I had proved so many people wrong. A lot of people had doubted me through my life, right from being at school, but I had proven to myself that I could do whatever I set out to achieve. I'm glad I hadn't listened to them. Or at least, I'm glad I managed to stop believing them. I had achieved what I had set out to do. And against all the odds, Michelle and I had thrived. We loved each other, and supported each other, and we had an amazing son – the light of our world.

My journey has been long and painful and filled with tribulations, but I have come to this point in my life where I can appreciate everything that happened. I believe that things have a way of working themselves out, and, clearly, the things I went through helped me to get to where I am today. This is my one and only life, and I am glad that this is how I'm living it now.

Sometimes, I like to wonder what might happen if I went back in time to talk to my younger self. I might tell him that everything will work out, that he will become someone amazing, that he will improve understanding around some important issues. I might tell him that he's become a success, with a beautiful wife and son, and a family that adores him. I might even tell him that he's going to meet the Royal Family one day, be in the same room as the Duchess of Cambridge, and shake hands with Prince William.

But I don't know if I'd want to ruin the journey for him.

ACKNOWLEDGEMENTS

Thanks to Michelle, whose support has helped me along this entire way. I wouldn't be doing what I am today without her. To Ethan, my beautiful son, who I am so proud of.

To Mum, Dad, and Kevin for always being there for me. My wonderful second family, my mother and father-in-law Janet and Tony, who really helped us during Michelle's depression. All the mad family from the Rhondda, and the extended family members. I honestly feel like I couldn't have made it without you guys.

My best mate of over thirty years, Jason Elwood, and his wonderful family, and of course all my friends; you know who you are, always in my life and keeping my spirits up. I have been blessed to have so many great people around me. The wonderful people of the Ogmore Valley who have always helped me and never judged me; thank you for supporting me in all the work I do and will always continue to do for the rest of my life.

The people I now call friends who have helped me in mental health: Dr Jane Hanley, who has given me the confidence, and Mental Health Matters Wales, who I have been proud to work with since my breakdown. To Dr Andy Mayers, Dr Raja Gangopadhyay, Dr Anna Machin, Dr Daniel Singley, Professor Ian Jones and Maternal Mental Health Alliance who have always supported the work I do with fathers.

The people who have helped me in my recovery including Zoe Piper, Sarah Lloyd, Pam Rossiter, Dave (Alcohol Team) and the National Health Service. And to the professionals who helped Michelle as well; we can't thank you enough.

To all the campaigners including good friends Ashley Curry, Pauline Mcpartland, Olivia Spencer, Helen Birch, Paul Scates, Rosey from PND Hour State of Mind, Elaine Hanzak, Charlotte Harding, IHV, and anyone I have forgotten who has shared my work on social media.

And all the countless people who I could write an entire book of thanks about – I couldn't have done this without all of you.

If you found this book interesting …
why not read this next?

Postpartum Depression
and Anxiety
The Definitive Survival and Recovery Approach

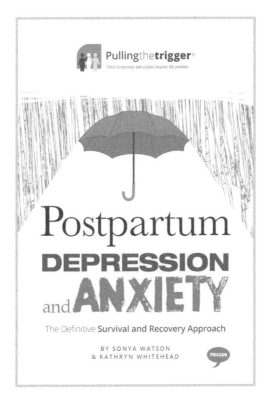

A refreshing, compassionate and user-friendly self-help book
to guide and support parents experiencing postpartum
depression and anxiety.

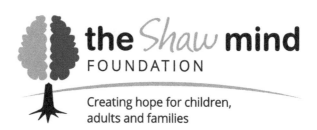

Sign up to our charity, The Shaw Mind Foundation
www.shawmindfoundation.org
and keep in touch with us; we would love to hear from you.

We aim to bring to an end the suffering and despair caused by mental health issues. Our goal is to make help and support available for every single person in society, from all walks of life. We will never stop offering hope. These are our promises.

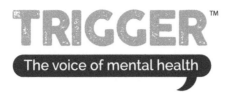

www.triggerpublishing.com

Trigger is a publishing house devoted to opening conversations about mental health. We tell the stories of people who have suffered from mental illnesses and recovered, so that others may learn from them.

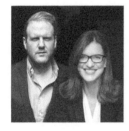

Adam Shaw is a worldwide mental health advocate and philanthropist. Now in recovery from mental health issues, he is committed to helping others suffering from debilitating mental health issues through the global charity he co-founded, The Shaw Mind Foundation. www.shawmindfoundation.org

Lauren Callaghan (CPsychol, PGDipClinPsych, PgCert, MA (hons), LLB (hons), BA), born and educated in New Zealand, is an innovative industry-leading psychologist based in London, United Kingdom. Lauren has worked with children and young people, and their families, in a number of clinical settings providing evidence based treatments for a range of illnesses, including anxiety and obsessional problems. She was a psychologist at the specialist national treatment centres for severe obsessional problems in the UK and is renowned as an expert in the field of mental health, recognised for diagnosing and successfully treating OCD and anxiety related illnesses in particular. In addition to appearing as a treating clinician in the critically acclaimed and BAFTA award-winning documentary *Bedlam*, Lauren is a frequent guest speaker on mental health conditions in the media and at academic conferences. Lauren also acts as a guest lecturer and honorary researcher at the Institute of Psychiatry Kings College, UCL.

Please visit the link below:

www.triggerpublishing.com

Join us and follow us...

@triggerpub

Search for us on Facebook